UNTIL THE COWS COME HOME

By
J.T. Blakemore

airleaf.com

ISBN: 1-60002-179-4

LETTERS OF REVIEW

"An amazing work – this book by J.T. I have read so many books in my career. But this one stands out as not only a compelling autobiography; not only delightfully fun to read; but also a bit of a tour de' force regarding what is possible with Closed Head Injuries (TBI). Joe not only tells us what is possible, he lives it.

I know Joe from working with him on some of the problems he has in living with the TBI. He's smart, tenacious and at times a bit irascible – but with an abiding faith in both God and himself to see him through. I'd recommend his book for any person with TBI, or involved with a person who has suffered such a trauma. But this is a delightful read for any of us – entertaining, funny, and motivating. It helps put our own, usually minor, problems into a different perspective. One of the best books I've had the pleasure to peruse for a very long time."

- Richard K. Lyon, Ph.D.
Clinical Psychologist
Tallahassee, Florida

"As you might imagine, I frequently receive copies of books written by survivors of brain injury and/or their families about how they have coped with devastating circumstances. All of them tell of incredible faith and determination to find meaning and strength to lead a productive life. Your book, however, told the story in a way that engaged me from start to finish and I was so moved that I purchased fifty copies for distribution from our office and fifteen copies to give to my family and friends.

In my opinion, your book *Until the Cows Come Home*, is a wonderful testimony to the ability of the human spirit to turn tragedy into a meaningful life the problems you experienced before the injury were enough for anyone to have to overcome, let alone trying to do it with a brain injury. I sincerely believe that your story provides a wonderful message of perseverance and hope that can inspire not just those who have a similar injury, but all those who are faced with difficult challenges and tribulations.

I wish you much success with the book and am happy to recommend it to anyone who appreciates a true, inspirational story told by the person who lived it."

- Ellie Kazuk
Brain Injury Association of Florida, Inc.
Pompano Beach, Florida

"Joe Blakemore is a resident of Tallahassee, Florida and a long-time survivor of a traumatic brain injury (TBI). His autobiography provides the reader with rare insight into the challenges, obstacles and frustrations of living a life with TBI. Throughout the book he discusses the sources of his strength including his faith, family, and friends who help him to continue to persevere on a daily basis. The book contains useful information that provides the reader with a better understanding of what it is like to function in a society during a time when health care professionals do not acknowledge or understand traumatic brain injury. J. T. Blakemore is commended for his accomplishment in writing this book and for his dedication to increase traumatic brain injury awareness and knowledge of health care professionals and others who work with individuals with a TBI.

On behalf of the program, I am pleased to make this book available to you. I feel confident it will assist all of us in our efforts to remove the obstacles, develop the supports, and better demonstrate the compassion and professional dedication, needed to assist individuals with disabilities to be accepted and fully integrated back into our communities."

- Thom DeLilla, Bureau Chief
Florida Department of Health, Brain and Spinal Cord Injury Program
Tallahassee, Florida

TABLE OF CONTENTS

To my son and daughter, Stephen and Erin, my loving wife Mary Nell, and every human being on this planet who has ever suffered brain damage, also known as TBI (traumatic brain injury).

FOREWORD

This book tells the story of an amazing man who sustained an injury and yet never let it define him. Make no mistake: Brain injury can be a life changing event, but Joe Blakemore should not be defined as just a person with a brain injury. He is that and much more.

Joe has seen quite a bit of adversity in his life, even before his automobile accident in 1963. From his years in an orphanage to his dreams of becoming a professional baseball player that were cut short by a severe knee injury, his life has been one of cruel ironies and continual adaptation. Don't get me wrong: He did not always cope with these challenges well, but through it all he has somehow managed to maintain his sense of humor. He has come a long way, and today this consummate storyteller is one of the most enthusiastic men you will ever meet. From not ever being expected to walk, talk, or see normally again, he has gone on to earn several college degrees, meet and marry his wife, and raise two children. So this book is not just for those with brain injuries. It can serve as an inspiration to all of us who have ever faced adversity and contemplated giving up.

Until quite recently, I was the supervisor for the helpline at the national office of the Brain Injury Association of America. That's how I met Joe Blakemore. Unhappy with the response he got from the Helpline staff, he asked to speak to the boss, and he got me. All he wanted was for us to change the workers' compensation system in Florida. And to tell him how to get better. And to find him a lawyer who was an expert in brain injury law. Unfortunately, climbing the ladder, so to speak, did not change the answer. I told him we could do one of the three things he asked for. He said, in so many words, that we were worthless. After he was done yelling at me, I told him that he could shoot the messenger as many times as he wanted, but the answer would not change. And so began our relationship: on the phone, he in Florida, me in Virginia. I have never met him in person, but I know him.

I have spoken about brain injury and what can happen following a brain injury with about 5,000 to 6,000 people on the average every year. I have heard stories about the impossible happening, both good and bad, and everything in between. People with brain injury are often misunderstood. They do not necessarily look "disabled" so many people think their "forgetfulness" is laziness, stupidity, or apathy. Once you have read this book, you will see for yourself that Joe is far from lazy, stupid or apathetic. In fact, he's an inspiration.

Joe and I have talked several times a year over the last five years, and I could hear the change in his cognition over time. He got better at finding the right words, and recalling previous conversations with only minimal help. This gives some insight into what is possible after a brain injury. When I first spoke with him, Joe was argumentative and saw the world with blinders on. He saw the world his way, and to him, it was the only way. If I contradicted him or tried to give him information to change his views, he became belligerent and would not even consider the idea that his world view might not be the only one. But over time I noticed that he began to listen to me.

I was interested in understanding how these improvements could occur more than thirty years after his original injury. That's when he told me he had started to write a book about his experiences. It is impossible to stress how great an accomplishment this book actually is. Having done cognitive therapy with people who are trying to return to work or school after their injury, I have seen up close and personal the process of redefining yourself in its aftermath. The process one goes through in brain injury rehabilitation can be a very personal and intense one. You have to take a long look at what you can and cannot do, and make serious decisions about the path your life will take, all while trying to understand things like why you can't do a simple word search puzzle when before your injury you could finish most of the Sunday crossword. Making the leap from there to deciding to write a book takes a great deal of self-confidence. This book has been a labor of love for Joe and a terrific challenge for him as well.

It became clear to me that the process of recalling events and writing them down was having a significant effect on Joe's cognition in other areas. To understand how important that is, one has to understand the basic assumptions about brain injury over the last twenty-five years. Back when Joe was injured, there was no rehabilitation for cognition. If you were injured in an accident, you received rehabilitation for your physical injuries, but nothing else. Even as recently as twenty years ago, there were only a handful of places that even attempted to rehabilitate people with brain injury. That is part of the reason why the Brain Injury Association (then called the National Head Injury Foundation) was founded. (Check out Appendix C in the back of this book for information about this and many other fine organizations.) The amount of information available to families up to that point was almost nonexistent. Today, a person can expect to receive inpatient therapy for both physical and cognitive deficits following an injury. Even so, until quite recently the basic assumption has been that a person makes the bulk of his or her improvements in the first year post injury. After that, progress seems to slow, and by the time two years have passed, there is not expected to be significant improvement.

What we are beginning to understand now more than ever before is how dynamic the brain really is. In the last few years, it has been discovered that the brain does indeed seem to generate new cells. It had always been assumed that you were born with all the brain cells you would need for your life. We also know that it might be possible for damaged brain cells to heal. There is still much left to understand about the workings of the brain, and how these new findings might be applied therapeutically, but it has changed the perspective of many researchers.

In Joe's case, however, there was no "magic bullet" or magic pill (though he did tell me he started to take Ritalin under a doctor's care, and that seemed to help him with paying attention to things). Even so, Joe undertook the "simple" task of starting to write down his life story. He soon discovered that the task was not as simple as he had originally estimated. So what made him continue? This is quite a complex, involved, long-term task, requiring the use of all kinds of memory – long-term, short-term, and sustained, to name a few. The world was telling him that what he was trying to do was much more difficult than he anticipated. At first, his usual response would be to react angrily, and stop the task. (For example, when he first came up with this idea and wanted me to tell him where to get his book published, my response was that he should focus on the book first, then figure out how to get it published as he got closer to completing it. I also told him we had no publishers calling us for books about brain injury, so the best I could do was give him a list of publishers we knew of that had published these types of stories before, or had published something about brain injury. His response was what I would call a less than friendly suggestion about what to do with my stupid association.) So what made him stick it out? Was it this decision that started to help him improve his memory and attitude? No one can say for sure.

What I definitely noticed over time was that as Joe worked on his book, his conversations with me became much more introspective and philosophical. As he progressed through his book he would call to get information or to bounce an idea off me. Even when I disagreed with what he was writing, he would now listen to my reasoning, and even though he still kept to his original assumptions, the process was much different than before.

I also noticed as he wrote the book that his perspective became much less egocentric. Instead of only wondering how something affected him, he started to ask questions about others. He started asking more about brain injury rehabilitation now versus twenty years ago, and wanted to know about the difficulties people with brain injuries have today. This was a radical change from previous conversations with him when his assumption was that if people get rehabilitation early for cognitive problems, the rest of their life is much easier. Just the process of starting to entertain the notion that you might have to change your perspective based on the information you receive from the world around you is often the start of personal improvement. That goes for all of us.

In the end, there is still a certain amount of the unknown in the progress Joe has made. I can say with some certainty that the process of writing his experiences down has helped him tremendously. This process is one he was heavily emotionally invested in. He wanted to see this through. That was part of why he was able to stick to this challenge more than he had to any other previous challenge. But what got him to start to see this as a challenge to be tackled? How did that "light bulb" come on in his head? That is the unknown, and continues to be the unknown in brain injury rehabilitation. But once that light bulb comes on, the ability to improve attitude, aptitude, and functioning improves dramatically.

In addition to illustrating that adversity can be overcome, this book offers several more specific things that I believe can be of great value. The first thing this book provides is a long-term view of brain injury. Many personal stories on brain injury today are about people who are three to five years post injury and are still learning to live with that injury. These books are important, no doubt. But what is not out there is a book about what happens ten or twenty years after the injury, a book that allows you to actually "get inside the head" of someone who has had to cope with this type of injury for the long term.

In 1960, more than half the people who sustained a severe brain injury died. The care and technology were just not there. More recent statistics for the CDC show that the mortality rate from brain injury seems to be around 20 to 25%. There are many more people living with brain injury today than there were just thirty years ago, so there is a big question as yet unanswered for society: What happens to someone who survives a brain injury in the long term? How do you learn to live with brain injury forever? Since there are no magic potions or panaceas, what we rely on is the experience of those who live it. These experiences are invaluable to others who are living with a brain injury who want to have some inkling, some little seed of an idea of what their life might be like in ten years, in twenty years. This book offers them a glimpse into that world.

No book will offer all the answers. No book will tell you exactly what will happen. But in this book are "nuggets" of useful information and insights. You have to decide which ones will be most valuable to you. You have to choose which nuggets you will keep, and which ones you will pass over. This book is full of nuggets—useful insights and anecdotes that describe adversity overcome, and, more specifically, life with a brain injury at a time when no one understood brain injury. It describes the challenge of getting help and of getting people to understand your experiences. It is a book about life, about challenges, and about the spirit of meeting a challenge—even one that lasts a lifetime.

I highly recommend writing down one's experiences to any reader who has sustained a brain injury. Whether or not these experiences become published as Joe's have been, the process itself might be part of an increased understanding of your injury as well as the first steps on a path that leads to living the life you are capable of living.

Life does go on after a brain injury. Just ask Joe Blakemore.

Gregory Ayotte has a B. A. in Psychology and is currently the program director for the Neurotrauma Registry, an online directory of brain and spinal cord injury programs. He is also the former director of information services for the Brain Injury Association of America. Mr. Ayotte writes this foreword not as an official endorsement from either organization, but as a friend and admirer of Mr. Blakemore's.

PREFACE

In my opinion, everyone should write a book about his or her life, for posterity if for nothing else. The simple therapy one gets from putting words on paper and making sense of it all is absolutely incredible, to say the least. I must admit though that some of the things I have been able to recall and have set down on these pages are a bit on the shocking side.

One of the many traits of brain damage is being given to excessive talking. I have also been told many times that I have a real need to explain things away. Someone asked me just the other day if I had a headache. After groping a bit, I blurted out what seemed to me to be a couple of misleading sentences. Finally, after attempting to correct the situation, I realized that a simple "yes" or "no" was all that that person was looking for.

If you or anyone else were to ask me how I'm doing on any given day, I would, in all probability, say I'm doing fine. Or I might just attempt to tell you my life story. Standing up, speaking up, and shutting up combined with saying exactly what you mean and meaning exactly what you say may sound a bit trite, but having the ability to do it plus the memory necessary for recall is priceless. Loquacious is the label that Vocational Rehabilitation hung on me in an attempt to describe that trait. They simply never quit.

I don't quit either. But during my attempted recovery from TBI, I could never have accomplished any of the many things I have accomplished without the ability to make decisions and sacrifices in the face of adversity. The Lord has given me the strength and peace of mind it takes to make the important decisions and sacrifices in my life. More than anything, I want people to realize that it is possible to overcome adversity of any kind, no matter how overwhelming it may seem at the time. If I can do it, so can you! So don't give up!

My story deals with more than overcoming adversity caused by TBI (believe me, that alone is more than enough to deal with), but if you picked up this book mainly to learn more about TBI, you may want to read appendices in the back of the book first. They include a great deal of basic information that you may find helpful. But once you've done that, I hope you'll get back to the "good stuff": my story, of course!

I often wonder exactly why I wrote this book. I remember suggesting to someone years ago that I had a lot to say about life in general and mine in particular. Whoever that person was, I believe he said something about me trying to make a silk purse out of a sow's ear. However, the real reason for my writing is that it seems to work wonders for my overall well-being. The more I think, the better I think, and the better I think, the better I write. And then there's that small voice deep inside of me that gently urges me to do it. I'm sincerely hoping that this book will be a big help to a few people and perhaps even a few more than that.

I have run into so much difficulty while working on this story. More times than I care to count, I thought I could not go on. Things like family problems and other personal problems like my poor health have caused many setbacks. At times it's as if "they're" trying to keep me from completing my work. Exactly who "they" are has not been that hard for me to figure out: the powers that be. But with the powers that be held at bay and with God's blessing in abundance, getting back to my work has been done and done and done again. And now it is done! Wow!

I feel a strong urge to quote the nineteenth century impressionist artist Renoir here. "One must, from time to time, attempt things that are beyond one's capacity." Perhaps the decision I made to write this book in the first place was beyond my capacity, but with the Lord's help, it was done. The opportunity for me to write at this time in my life is truly wonderful! I have been blessed in all of my attempts to write my story and I do believe you will be blessed for having read it!

An ancient Hebrew sage once said, "Of the making of many books there is no end..." (Ecclesiastes 12:12). Here's hoping there is room for one more.

ACKNOWLEDGMENTS

I'd like to thank a few people and organizations for helping me to accomplish this writing: VSA Arts of Florida, The Able Trust, First Florida Pooled Trust, Childserv, the Brain Injury Association of America and its Florida chapter, and Houston Seals. I am also very grateful to Greg Ayotte and two of my neighbors, Jim St. John and Sherman Sasser, who were willing to read portions of my manuscript and offer encouragement. Jan Bevan, an accomplished author in her own right, put me in touch with a professional editor. Barb Abelhauser (editpro@yellowhammer.com) has proven to be a dedicated professional with profound editorial skills. Barb has edited my work from beginning to end and is one super human being. My Lord Jesus Christ has definitely brought my cows home once again!

"To thine own self be true."

—William Shakespeare

INTRODUCTION

My name is Joseph Thomas Blakemore, Joe for short, or J.T.—even shorter. Many TBI survivors would agree that shorter is usually better. I was born on July 1, 1941 in Colorado Springs, Colorado. Just like many of you, no doubt about it, I have been caught up in adversity since birth. The one thing that might set us apart is the fact that I am a survivor of brain damage and all the problems that come with it.

Living our lives and overcoming obstacles beyond the norm can be overwhelming. Seemingly everyone has a tale to tell along these lines. That fact has always made me feel somewhat insignificant. Realizing my own significance in life has not been at all easy for me. I suspect many of you feel the same way. But I have become convinced that one's background, especially in the areas of education and faith, is the key to overcoming adversity of any kind.

At the risk of sounding like one big crybaby (believe me, I have cried out to God many times in my life and I'm not ashamed to admit it), I have had what some might say was my fair share of hard times. But no matter how tough life gets for me, I have always been of the understanding that someone else has it a lot tougher.

Some of what I consider to be the more serious difficulties I have faced in my life include a broken home and its aftermath; living with relatives, in foster homes, and in a place called the Lake Bluff Orphanage; and, later, the failed reconciliation attempts between my mother and father.

Then, in 1962, I injured my left knee to a point beyond repair at that time. (Isn't it amazing how far medical science has come since then? The old adage "a day late and a dollar short" seems to have fit me fine for much of my life. Perhaps you can identify with that to some extent yourself.)

It was in the following year that I suffered brain damage, also known as TBI (traumatic brain injury), in an automobile accident. I was told that I was lucky to be alive, and that would be true even today. (Medical science has not gotten quite that far yet.).

I have also experienced third degree burns over one third of my body, prostate cancer (the aggressive type), and two types of skin cancer: squamous cell carcinoma and melanoma. The melanoma involved the removal of a not-so-small piece of my favorite shoulder.

I believe God is using me for his purpose, and I try not to question that. I definitely don't believe in luck. Seven years after my near fatal accident, and only by the grace of God, I found the answer to all of the adversities in my life. I have found peace and purpose in my life regardless of all of the roadblocks I have encountered along the way.

This story of mine is not only about overcoming TBI, it's about overcoming all the adversities in life—big and small. I did it and so can you. Anyone can. If that sounds like I believe that I have all of the answers pertaining to life's hardships, let me assure you that I believe I do have more than a few. More importantly, though, I know who has *all* of the answers.

In the end, one might say my story is simply about living life. I hope you enjoy reading it half as much as I have enjoyed writing it. May we all find opportunity through adversity. Believe me, it's always there.

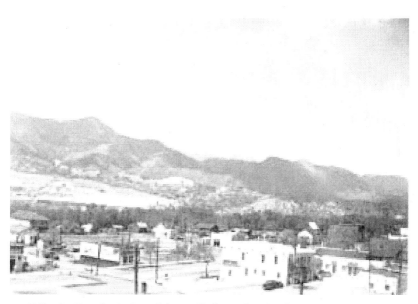

Pike's Peak & Rockies, Colorado Springs, May 1941

CHAPTER 1

A True Wanderlust

I'm not going to start my story by telling you about my auto accident in 1963. Instead, I'll begin with background information. Believe me, the past experiences of any head injury survivor play a key role in his or her recovery. My story begins with my father and my mother only because without them, obviously, I myself would not exist.

My biological parents were both born in Iowa in 1916. My father was a very bright man, although irresponsible and immature. He never did grow up. He was small in stature, standing only about five foot seven at best, yet strength was written all over him. He had jet black hair and a personality that many women of that day found irresistible.

He was an extremely functional illiterate with little education. He loved to drink beer, ride "hogs" and Indians (motorcycles, that is), and raise hell. He really didn't care much about life—his or anyone else's. My father was a Hell's Angel before the Hell's Angels ever were.

My mother had been the valedictorian of her high school class of 1934 in Corydon, Iowa. She was a very intelligent person—more than simply bright. She was a fine looking woman—thin and golden-haired, but she had been born "behind the eight ball," as she often liked to say, into a very poor Iowa dirt farmer's family. She said she had been thrown to the wolves—thrust headlong into the Roaring Twenties and the Great Depression.

Although her intellect served her well throughout her life, my mother's heart got her into trouble. She married my father three times. My parents were both persistent people when it came to their quest for the American dream, to say the least. They were married for the first time in 1936. They actually met and got married on the same day, and neither one of them missed the following work-day. A story about the affair appeared in the Des Moines Register, in the human interest column. However, the version of the story that I claimed to be the absolute truth for most of my life went something like this:

Georgia Ruth Barnes was working as a waitress in a small restaurant in Des Moines. She was becoming more and more discouraged with her life with every passing day. She had done exceptionally well as a student and would have jumped at the chance to study beyond high school, but she had long since accepted the fact that she was dirt poor. She began feeling trapped and frustrated with her overall situation. The idea of a knight in shining armor began to dance through her mind. Early one morning she stood near the cash register, counting her change. Suddenly there was a great deal of excitement in the air. The roar of her armor-clad knight's steel horse as it came crunching through the heavily graveled parking lot replaced her frustration, and she welcomed the thought of a new dance. The moment he swaggered through the door she knew him. In less time than it takes most folks to order two eggs over easy and a cup of coffee, Ruth (as she insisted everyone call her as she did not, at all, care for her first name) said yes to Donald Arthur Blakemore's proposal of marriage.

This story had been lost in my damaged brain for years, and was only brought back to my memory recently and unexpectedly after a rather long conversation with my half sister. I guess I had come to believe it in time because I was always looking for the best in my parents. Isn't everyone? My own insistence on believing whatever I wanted to believe along with some input from an overactive imagination allowed me to attach a romantic twist to their story. Donald Arthur as a knight in shining anything would be a real twist. I think one of the hardest things for anyone to do in life is admit that his or her parents were wrong about anything.

Now I'll tell you the rest of my story from the point of view of a true wanderlust. (My mother told me that my father often called me his little wanderlust.)

My father quit school in the early 1930's. At the age of sixteen, he rode his motorcycle from Iowa to California and joined the CCC, the Civilian Conservation Corps, where he became a short order cook. The CCC was one of the earliest New Deal programs during the Great Depression.

Somehow my father managed to become a chef, a highly skilled cook, and was very good at his trade. He never did learn to read or write much, but when it came to the preparation of food, he was exceptionally good. Some time after their first marriage in 1936, my parents moved to Colorado. They were always moving. Ruth often remarked that Don could not stay in one place for very long. He went to work as head chef in the old Antlers Hotel in late 1939.

I have my father to thank for my first big shock in life (circumcision notwithstanding), at the age of two. He was a real motorcycle buff in the late thirties and early forties, and owned this big 1937 Indian that he loved more than life itself. One afternoon when my mother was not home, he sat me on the gas tank of that bright and shiny Indian and told me to hang on. Believe me, I did—for dear life. He cranked it on and we were off. It was one wild and windy ride for a two-year-old! But the first time was definitely not the charm.

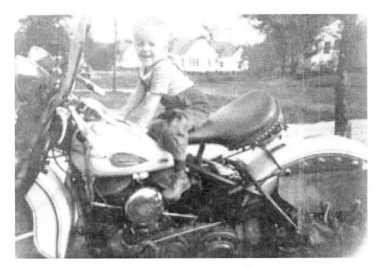

Me on the new "hog"

I was not as frightened as I was thrilled. I was so excited, in fact, that I wet my shorts. (I had been out of diapers for some time.) The force of the acceleration pressed my small body back against his large Harley Davidson belt buckle. My short, bare legs were dangling below the gas tank and just above the spark plug wire leading to that big Indian's head. The shocking sensation that followed almost knocked us both off the bike. It didn't, however, and neither of us was seriously hurt, I guess.

My mother told me that story so many times that I actually think I have a vague recollection of the incident. I have often wondered what Sigmund Freud (who was, in my opinion, the height of misguided intellect) might have done with that little story.

In addition to Don's other shortcomings, it seems that he had an extraordinarily hard time dealing with success. He left his job in Colorado Springs in 1943. That was the beginning of a muddy road for me, for sure.

It was after leaving his job at the Antlers Hotel that I believe the first divorce took place. I am sure that the trip back to the Chicago area had a good deal to do with my mother's decision to leave Sir Donald. Try and picture a pregnant woman, a two-year-old child (me), and our family dog, all riding on a brand-new Harley Davidson motorcycle. My father, of course, was at the controls. Well armored he was, wearing his black motorcycle boots, a brown leather jacket, and a matching brown leather aviator's cap with goggles. Most everything the man had on was First World War vintage. Believe me, I've seen the pictures and he looked a lot like the infamous Red Baron, the Germans' ace flyer of that war.

Our dog, a fine little mutt named Skipper, perhaps would have been more appropriately named Snoopy, at least for that trip. He rode in the saddle bags of the new bike for the entire journey back to the Big Windy. I don't have the slightest conscious recollection of the trip, but I was told about it many times. Apparently we ran into some stormy weather: wind, rain, and muddy roads. My mother was not really happy with the mode of travel in the first place. She said we were all soaked to the bone by the time we got to Cedar Rapids, Iowa.

I don't know how my father ever managed to separate himself from that 1937 Indian. One of his brothers still talks about how much Don loved that machine. By the way, all of my father's siblings—two brothers and two sisters—lived long, full, prosperous lives. Ruth often said the rest of the Blakemores were normal people.

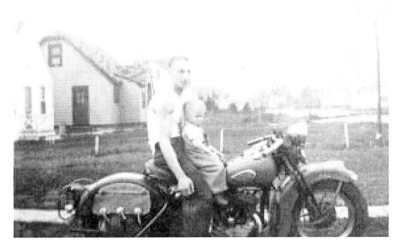

Don Blakemore, his old Indian and me. 1943

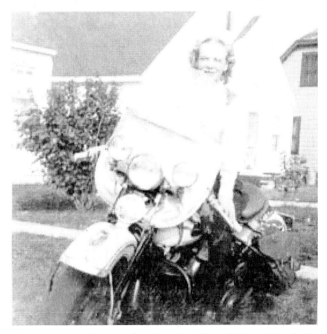

Ruth Blakemore on her new Harley Davidson back in Illinois.

The story my mother told about the new Harley he bought just before our stormy trip back to Chicago in 1943 was an interesting one. My mother wanted a new car, "like normal people," she said. Well, my father told her this wild story about how he had come to realize just how dangerous motorcycles could actually be. He went on to tell her how he had almost been killed a day or two before. His big Indian had gone into what he told her was a high-speed wobble. It took two other guys, and both of them were riding brand-new "hogs", one on each side of his bike, to pull him out of it. The fact that he was still alive was solely due to the cruising capability and the new engineering and safety features of those new Harley Davidsons. Without them he would have never made it home alive. The Harley Davidson motorcycle company had really put safety first, he told her, and the new ride was one of true comfort. He simply had to have one! You know my mother caved, and he got his new hog.

By the time I was in high school I had the high-speed wobble story down to a science. And I had found out that the wobble was actually a real problem with the old Indian motorcycles. The science came in due to the fact that the wind pressure or draft from the two hogs had helped to stabilize the Indian.

Even though Ruth had seemingly given in to his story, she really wanted a new car. "At least we would have all been dry. You know, Joe, you were sandwiched between us and I did keep you dry for a good while. I had the back of Don's leather jacket pulled over your head. I tried to press up as close as I could in my condition but you still got soaked. Motorcycles are for the birds." Then she added with that all-knowing, all-understanding, very comforting smile of hers, "Your father was mud from head to toe." It was my mother's heart that got us all wet, and I'm sure she new it.

I don't recall that long, wet, and at times very muddy trip back to Illinois. Stormy weather, wind, rain, and mud, even getting soaked to the bone has never bothered me one bit. On the contrary, I love it!

They were divorced and remarried within ninety days of this stormy trip. (This first divorce remains unsubstantiated due to poor record keeping. All the conversations I had with my mother over the years lead me to believe it took place in July, 1943.) My mother told me that she thought she had made a big mistake. From what I understand, our parents were remarried just in time for my sister's birth.

Shortly after their second marriage came a new house in Round Lake, Illinois, my baby sister, and a new restaurant owned and operated by the head chef himself. My family was on a roll. Shoot, I even won a baby contest in our new community (best all-around baby). All right! All these great things took place in less than two years' time. Things were looking extra good once more.

One not-so-minor detail was being overlooked, however. It seems that along with the new restaurant came the other woman. Ruth confronted Donald about his extramarital affair (or perhaps affairs) in 1945, and he ran like a well-hooked blue marlin. I didn't see him or his iron horse again for almost a decade.

The second divorce, however, did not take place until 1948. My father's whereabouts had been unknown for some time. We were always told that Daddy had just run away from home one day. We always seemed to have the hope that Ruth's knight in shining armor, our father, would come swaggering through the door once more. That never did happen. However, there would be a third marriage and reconciliation attempt.

While staying with an aunt and uncle in Fairview, Illinois, my mother heard, for the first time in at least five years, from her ex-husband, my runaway father. In short order, she was on her way to Miami. Shortly after that they were remarried. The big reconciliation attempt, of which my sister and I both became a part, proved not to be our dream come true. It was simply one big flop. Seeing my mother cry and watching my estranged father staggering, stumbling, and swearing at the world bothered me a great deal. I really believe that if my father had struck my mother in my presence at that time, I would have attempted to kill him. Really! Then Wobbly Don, the runaway father, did it again.

The cowardly men who leave their offspring hanging in this world should themselves be hanged by specific parts of the male anatomy until dead. Politically incorrect, I'm sure, and graphically strong language coming from a licensed minister of the gospel, true. Perhaps, however, it's to be expected coming from an ex-marine with an axe to grind and some serious chopping to do.

My mother got the house, which was not much of a house to begin with. I got a really nice little Doberman puppy that was soon to be too much of a dog. My sister didn't get much, as usual.

TBI can be more than hard to deal with at times. About three years into my battle to regain some sort of normal existence, seemingly out of nowhere many of my past experiences began to flash through my mind. These flashbacks never appeared to be related to anything in particular, and remained random in their occurrences. After a while I learned to enjoy my flashbacks. I was able to find humor in this sort of thing most of the time. Some of these random thoughts would repeat over and over again just like a stuck record on an old record player. I found that if I concentrated on the repeated thought, most of the time a couple of extremely clear and precise sentences would follow. Many times, though, only clear and precise nonsense followed. On one of these occasions, the following came to my mind in its entirety (although I could not use a pencil at the time, some years later I wrote it down and even gave it a name):

Trees!
(By me, J.T.)

There are just about as many trees in this old world as there are men, but seldom am I to see a man with the roots of a tree!

My father worked in Miami Beach at the Kenilworth Hotel in the late fifties. He was the head chef for a famous radio personality for years, or so I have been told. Even though I really didn't know where my father was at the time, it has always made me feel good to *believe* that little story about him, anyway. Thinking along genetic lines, the more good things I know about my father (and believe me, I keep looking), the better I feel. In all honesty though, I have never had much, if any, unselfish interest in him. On the other hand, simply being aware of the fact that he had no apparent interest in me has been a really sore spot in my life.

Not only did he refuse to help my mother in any way with the support of their two children, but also he became a hopeless alcoholic. During the late forties and early fifties he was called Wobbly Don in the local bars. To this day, you can go into one of those bars in Northwest Miami and order a drink that bears that name. Wobbly Don's foolproof way of dealing with life's problems (remaining blind and oblivious to them) apparently led him to see adversity as something that was impossible to overcome. He also managed to father at least two other children that I know of—one younger and one older than my sister and I. We have never met either of them.

My mother was truly a master when it came to dealing with the adversity she faced in her life. I can't say that she ever completely overcame any of it, but she did a masterful job of dealing with it for the most part. On the other hand, though, in the mind of this writer (her son, her knight in shining armor's wanderlust), the difference between dealing with adversity and overcoming it is a profound one.

By 1955 we were in a brand-new house in North Miami Beach. Mother had a new husband and we had a stepfather. He did not care much for my dog. They soon found a new home for it. My mother said I would get over it and that one day I would understand.

Ruth seemed to become a little more agnostic with every passing year. She had been raised a rip-roaring Baptist. Those were her very words. You could say I was taught about God at her knee. My mother had decided by the time I was born that if there really was a God, her son was bound to need divine help with his life sooner or later. So, due to her uncertainty, on the twenty-eighth of July, 1941, I became a member of the cradle roll of the Trinity Evangelical Church in Colorado Springs, Colorado. I was twenty-eight days old and I had already been dedicated to Jesus Christ. (No, I don't have the T-shirt, but I did find the certificate.)

Even though she said she was not sure about the existence of God, my mother always expressed a steadfast hope in his existence. I can't say that she ever accepted Christ in her life, but I will never say she did not know the Lord, either. God is the judge, not I. One thing this old wanderlust is sure of, however, is that he would have liked to have found out about that dedication ceremony long before he did. My mother was right about one thing for sure: I have definitely needed an abundance of divine help in my life. A wanderlust without God is definitely something I would not care to be!

CHAPTER 2

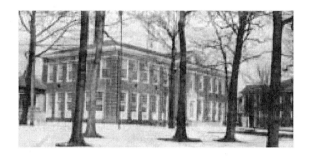

Institutionalized!

The formative years of my life, from ages four to twelve, were spent living somewhere other than with my father. I stayed either in foster homes, with relatives, or in a place called the Lake Bluff Orphanage during that entire period. I didn't deal very well with adversity during those early years of my life. I am convinced that my childhood and misspent youth ultimately led the way to my accident in 1963. (We definitely will arrive at the scene of my accident. Really.)

I started my grade school education in 1947 at Westmont Elementary School in Westmont, Illinois. At that time, I was six and one-half years old and living in a foster home outside of Chicago in Blackhawk Heights, a nearby suburban community. I was living with V.L. Engstrom, his wife Pauline, daughter Mary Jo, and a great family dog named Pudge, who rapidly became my best friend. (Pudge was a setter/pointer mix, and the best rock retriever I have ever known, bar none. I would often throw stones for hours and that dog would seldom lose one.)

The Engstroms had a fine home, a real home, and they gave me the best family life I had ever known, bar none again!

However, in the long term, things would not work out for me there, either. The Engstroms (Ma and Pa, as they liked to be called, by me anyway) wanted to adopt me, but didn't think they could give both my sister and me the home we needed. My mother was steadfast in her decision not to split us up for good if she could possibly find another way. She did. She found the Lake Bluff Orphanage in Lake Bluff, Illinois.

My mother always said she had to tell the people at Lake Bluff a little white lie about the Engstroms. I gained a full understanding of what she meant only recently. My mother felt that she had a better chance of getting us placed in the orphanage if she led the authorities to believe that the Engstroms were trying to take both of her children away from her. She was convincing even though, in reality, I had been living with the Engstroms much longer than my sister had. My sister had been in more foster homes than I had, but ultimately we both spent two years institutionalized.

In the summer of 1951 I became a member of Wadsworth 1 in the upstairs dorm of Wadsworth Hall. I had no idea who Mr. Wadsworth was, and I still don't. Sorry. I do know that the main building of the LBO was where the meanest old man alive lived— the Monster, Dean-of-the-Whole-World. (I remember one time when the Monster paddled the little red-headed demon that lived downstairs. That kid swore he would never again own a wallet like the one he had in his pocket on that day in 1951. The poor little brat had the impression of a horse head on his butt for a week.) I stayed away from the main building and tried to be as good as I

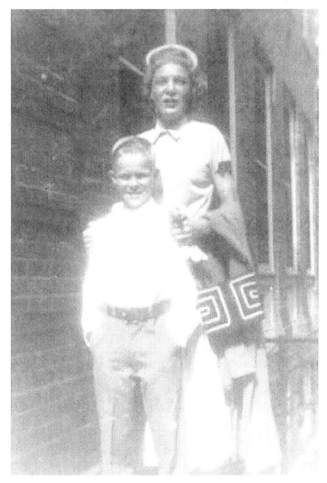

Mom & Joe on the steps of the Lake Bluff Orphanage, 1951.

possibly could at all times, for sure. I could not stand the idea of having to go see the Monster, the Mean Dean.

After the move was made, like all the rest of the children in the orphanage we were enrolled in Lake Bluff Elementary School, where I started the third grade. I had already gone through second grade twice. Due to all the moving around we did, getting though the second grade had become a big problem.

The school in Lake Bluff was within walking distance of Our Good Old LBO, as most all of us orphanage kids insisted on calling our home. This name was not particularly pleasing to the folks in the main building whom we always called the Old Farts. (They never had a clue that we called them that as far as we knew.)

Soon many of my classmates, kids from out in the community, were coming home with me to see where I lived and what it was like to live in the orphan home. One LBO counselor remarked, "This kid is like Will Rogers." I guess he meant I never met a kid I didn't like. I really didn't have a clue at the time. I thought he had made a mistake, and I was quick to correct him: "Roy, not Will!"

My sister never did adapt to living in the orphanage, or to any part of our ordeal, for that matter. We were very close and we both felt a strong affection one for the other. It was so hard for us to understand why we were always being separated. During the time we lived in Lake Bluff we did see each other more often than we ever had before although she lived with the girls in her dorm and I of course lived in the boys' dormitory.

My little sister sure was a beautiful little girl, and she has gone on to raise three beautiful children of her own. Her life hasn't been easy, but she knows the value of it all. We still talk about the early years and how we would have liked things to have been. We agree that all either one of us ever truly wanted was to be loved and to

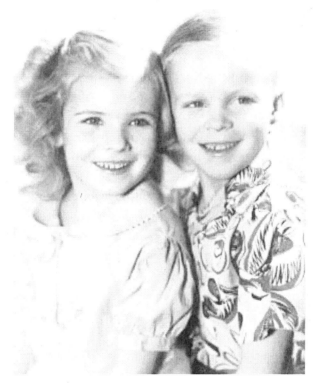

Joey and Judy before LBO, 1947.

know that we could love someone back who would still be in our lives tomorrow. Even though we have both had to go our separate ways in life there still remains a very strong bond between us.

I remember one of my friends from school. After he walked home with me one afternoon, he asked one of our dorm parents if I could spend the weekend at his house. Well, about a week later all the arrangements had been made, and on the following Friday I walked home from school with him, my toothbrush in my pocket.

I was shocked! I simply did not realize anyone lived in a house that big. He had his own room, a big black and tan dog, and lots of toys and games, plus two of the nicest parents I had ever met. As if that wasn't enough, the kid even had his own ant colony. Obviously, this kid had it even better than David and Ricky Nelson. (That was an afterthought that occurred to me about a year later, after Ozzie and Harriet, the ideal American family of the day, made its way onto the TV set of Wadsworth 1.) Man, what a house! And man, what a family!

I was really thrown for a loop, and had instant mixed emotions to say the least, when I was told by a counselor a couple of days later that this kid's parents had called the orphanage and requested my mother's address and phone number. They wanted to talk to her. His parents actually wanted to adopt me.

I could tell my friend didn't like hearing me say no to the adoption offer. His parents seemed to understand. He would always tell me about all of the fun we could have if I would just let his parents adopt me. Everything would be great. It might have been, at that. Of course, I would talk to him almost every day at school. I even stayed overnight at his house a couple of times after that.

Over the years, the "adopt me" situation came up many times. Even though it was a bit frightening, I had a lot of faith and trust in my mother and her promise to keep us all together. She always did just that. At any rate, I never wanted to leave my sister or my mother behind. At that time in my life I would have never considered being adopted. I was prepared to fight adoption kicking and screaming all the way. You know, "until the cows come home." My mother used to say that all the time. I guess that's why I say it. I loved my mother and her cows, not to mention the idea of our own home and our family being all together—all the good stuff.

However, I have often thought, "What if...?" What would adoption have meant in my life? Of course, I'll never know now. I don't even remember all of the people involved. I only wish I could be adopted now. (Just kidding.)

I think I had better explain something before confusion takes over. Back in the fifties the Lake Bluff Orphanage was a place for children who either had no parents at all or had only one parent who was having a difficult time supporting them, which was our situation.

Most of the children in the LBO who didn't have any parents at all were infants, and they were all looked after in what was called Baby Fold. Baby Fold was the source of one of the most dreaded chores any of us, members of Wadsworth 1, ever had to do. Each winter morning, one of us had to get up at 4:30. We would then walk through the deep snow, often in below freezing temperatures and sometimes in blizzard-like conditions. We had to go approximately 100 yards across the large playground to Baby Fold, pick up bags of dirty, wet diapers, and then carry them back over to the laundry. Many times I had to drag a bag of diapers along behind me with yet another one slung over my favorite shoulder. Most of the time, my total load was heavier than I was.

Finally, I would arrive at the ever-so-loud, ever-so-warm laundry building. Boy, oh boy, was it cold outside! The warmth of the steamy, smelly laundry felt more than a little bit welcome after trudging through snowdrifts, three feet deep and deeper. The worst days were the blizzard days or the days when "the Hawk" was out. (For those of you who have never lived in the Chicago area, the Hawk is the wind coming off Lake Michigan on an icy-cold day.) The days of the Hawk were definitely the coldest days of my young life.

I have never forgotten the one-armed man who ran that laundry. He always seemed to be so appreciative, so happy to see me. He always made me feel like I was a really big man. I would always leave his laundry with a super feeling, a feeling of real accomplishment. That one-armed man always had something good to say, and he never failed to mention God. Adversity overcome?

He was the first person that I ever heard telling me that Jesus was the son of God. I took this information back to the other boys. It soon became the topic of many unresolved arguments.

I by no means want this to sound like a cop-out to you, the reader, but I have forgotten many of the details of my orphanage experiences. I could make up stuff, but I won't because this is supposed to be a true story. I'm not going to give the least bit of consideration to my overactive imagination, I promise!

I do vividly remember bits and pieces of one particularly wonderful experience in the summer of 1953. I'm going to try some reconstruction here, so hang on.

The counselors took all of us, some seven or ten boys who had not been given the opportunity to go home for the seemingly very long and hot summer, on a canoe trip. What a trip! Our adventure began in Wisconsin, very close to Minnesota, at a place called the Dells. Anyway, I remember one of the big boys telling me that when we got close to Minnesota we would know it because everyone there talked funny. Well, since I could not understand a word one old man was saying when we first climbed into our canoes (anyone over the age of thirty-five looked old to me back then), I figured we were in Minnesota already.

For days we paddled our canoes through one lake after another. Most of the time we would have a late lunch. The daylight seemed to last and last. Boy, was it hot! At night we would all sleep on a small island if one was available or on the shore if we had to. After paddling a canoe all day, most of us didn't care *where* we slept, just as long as we *did*. By the time it got dark, sleep was pretty darn welcome.

Thinking back to spending nights on those small islands reminds me of one very disturbing night, for sure. As usual, the daylight seemed to go on and on, but finally the sunset came along, and it started to get dark in one big hurry. Shadows were dancing here and there, playing tricks with my eyesight. We were all spreading out our bedrolls or sleeping bags if we had them. I did not. I spied this big round thing that looked to me like it would be softer to sleep on than the hard ground would be. As a matter of fact, I saw four of these things lying fairly close to one another. I slid two of them under my thin little pillow and didn't think any more about it. Bad move. The two objects, as I found out very early the next morning, were called "cow pies." Believe me, those so-called cow pies had begun to smell like what they really were after I had slept quite comfortably on them all night. Stink, stank, stunk!

You might be thinking the same thing I was thinking back then. How did cows get on the island, anyhow? But then, if you're like me, you think a bit more, and with the help of the counselors you figure it all out. When the sun came up that morning, we could see a large raft tied securely to a tree on the opposite shore. One of those funny-talking Minnesota or Wisconsin farmers (it hardly mattered—they all sounded funny to me) would ferry his cattle back and forth from the mainland on that raft.

No, finding that out didn't do all that much for my embarrassment, but I was glad to find out that those farmers didn't have flying cows. That was what one of the other boys had tried to tell me, and I did give it some genuine consideration at that. I'm absolutely certain that he had given that idea a good bit of consideration himself. You bet! Flying cows and bombs away!

Our fantastic adventure came to an end in Rock Island, Illinois at the foot of Starved Rock. Starved Rock—what a story, and what a site. The Legend of Starved Rock is about American Indians and a battle in 1769 between two indigenous tribes of that area. The 125-foot-tall sandstone butte was named Starved Rock after the Illiniwek Indians chose starvation instead of surrendering to the Ottawa and the Potawatomi Indians. One counselor said the moral of the story was that some things are worth dying for. Another counselor said it was better to die by starvation than to be tortured to death. The Legend of Starved Rock, as told to us by the counselors, planted seeds of thought in all of our young minds, no doubt. The story, told to us at its actual site, was a great way to end our canoe trip.

The whole trip was a wonderful experience for an almost twelve-year-old boy in 1953. It would be great to be able to remember it all, I'm sure. Greater still, I would love to do it all again.

All in all, I stayed in Our Good Old LBO for two very long (and sometimes seemingly very short) years. I have no idea what it cost my mother, financially or emotionally, to keep us in that place. Evidently she thought it was the best she could do at the time. I remember asking her how long we were going to have to stay there. She gave me that all-knowing, all-understanding, very comforting smile of hers and said, "Well, Joe, it might just be until the cows come home."

Again, I simply cannot remember everything that happened back then. I know that in light of all that has happened in my life since those early days it's not going to be easy finding any of the stuff I'm looking for in these extremely cluttered salvage rooms of my mind, although I must admit stumbling and rummaging around in these junkyards is great fun and games, for sure. Some of the junk up here sure could use a good cleaning! And I thought that fancy drug Ritalin was going to get rid of these darn cobwebs. There are still a bunch of them up here. Strange as it no doubt sounds to you, I can remember my experiences with cow pies sooner than I can with concepts such as pi squared and the like.

Anyway, I'm going to try my best to remember, and I really do feel more than a little bit inspired to do this work, so please read on and let me do all the rummaging and stumbling that is necessary. With the Lord's help, even the necessary cleaning will be done. No question about it.

If you'd like to learn more about my stay at LBO from the adults' point of view, take a look at Appendix D. I think you'll find it very interesting. I certainly did, after all these years!

The time came for me to leave Our Good Old LBO. My mother simply could not meet the costs any longer. (She had been working as a waitress in a restaurant for six consecutive years. One night in 1953 it burned to the ground.)

Saying goodbye to the LBO was not all that easy for me. I really had grown very accustomed to living in that place in a relatively short period of time. On the other hand, the idea of Mom, apple pie and the American dream were very appealing to me. Mom and her cows.

My stay in the Lake Bluff Orphanage was a bittersweet experience overall. However, I believe that's where many of my life's most important foundations were set. Honesty, respect, compassion, fairness and a firm and unflappable belief in God are only a few of those important building blocks. I guess my love for the daily surprises and excitement of simply being a part of Wadsworth 1 and Our Good Old LBO gave me a good feeling about myself. I know one thing for sure: Most all of the boys living in Wadsworth 1 during that period felt as though they were having a great time. But at the same time we all knew we were missing something. I can only speak for myself when I tell you that living there was a paradoxical experience. For me it truly was, indeed.

Home is where the heart is, as the saying goes. Nothing in my life, except for God, of course, could possibly be more absolutely true as far as I'm concerned. Home is definitely where my heart has always wanted to be.

Although my broken home experience and my early years had given me my first taste of extreme adversity in life, it was certainly not my last. Many years later I found myself faced with hard times that appeared to be never-ending. Living in an orphanage was small potatoes compared to living with TBI. With TBI there was absolutely no silver lining in sight, but my orphanage experience taught me to never stop looking for one.

CHAPTER 3

Redemption—Not!

I know beyond a doubt that my love for the game of baseball began at Our Good Old LBO. Due to the constant physical competition there, I soon realized my speed and athletic ability and believed it to be my birthright. I became convinced at a young age that that ability alone would be my redemption for all of the woes of life. By the time I was in my late teens, baseball had become my secret ambition, a covert operation of sorts. Unfortunately, baseball as a priority in my life had to be moved to dead last, put on the back burner so to speak, all too often.

I remember finding a book that looked to be a bit worse for wear in the Wadsworth 1 rec. room. (At the time, I never made the connection between "rec. room" and "recreation room." I honestly thought they called it the rec. room because we always made such a big wreck of the place every time they let more than two or three of us in there at any one time.) Anyway, the book I found was a fat, slightly worn-out paperback with a red and black cover. I can almost see that old book now. I tried to read that paperback on more than one occasion. One of the older boys said it was Babe Ruth's autobiography. I did not have a clue as to what that meant. All I really needed to know was that the Babe had lived in an orphanage once, too. From that day on I was positive that the Babe was right there in Lake Bluff with me. I was absolutely, positively certain I would play ball forever.

What a life and what a dream. I'll share something else with you: I believe in angels, and it may well be that the Babe has been with me all of my life. (Not that Babe Ruth was an angel during his life any more than I have been in mine.) You might say I have always had an angel in my outfield!

After I left the orphanage in 1953, my love for the game of baseball never died. But when you're being moved "from pillar to post" it's very hard to become involved in much of anything. Finally, during the relatively short time I spent in the Miami area from 1952 to '58, I did have the opportunity to become involved, on my own, in Little League, Pony League, Babe Ruth League and PAL League. I even played for the Elks club.

The coach of the 1956 Elks club baseball team will be in my thoughts until the day I die. The man was in his sixties at the time and he was one of those people in my life that I could not ignore even if I wanted to. Of course, it was not possible for very many young men my age to ignore this guy. He looked like an old rosin bag with a personality. He had started playing baseball back in 1909 and he would tell you in a Miami millisecond that he had forgotten to stop. He was the kind of man that would have been very pleased to find out that someone had called him an old rosin bag behind his back. His name was Cap Gowdy and I soon became convinced that Cap knew more about baseball than the man who invented the game in 1839. (Abner Doubleday usually gets credited with the genesis of baseball in Cooperstown, New York.) Of course Cap Gowdy would have never deliberately suggested anything like that, but anything I ever wanted to know about how to play the game Cap knew, and then some.

One day after a sand lot-type practice game, I overheard him referring to me as the Flying Dutchman. I think the reference was more about my blond hair hanging out from under my hat than my ability to play ball like Honus Wagner. Anyway, hearing that gave me enough confidence to ask him if he thought I had what it took. The big smile that stretched across his weathered face was answer enough for me, but it was what Cap said that haunts me to this day. "Blakemore, if you stay healthy you will definitely play baseball." I loved the game.

I really loved to learn, as well. The truth of the matter is that I liked school, but as soon as I would get really interested, there was sure to be something going on at home. (Even during my LBO days there always seemed to be way too much going on. I was learning a lot about some very useful things, but very little about how to learn or how to study. My kid sister, eight years old at the time, told her dorm parents at Lake Bluff that there were too many people there. She may have been correct in her assessment.)

My security was always uncertain. What a drag. It just always seemed to me to be too late to care about the classroom. I knew that I was way ahead of other kids my age in many ways. So what if most of them could spell, read, write, and count better than I could? In all too many cases I felt I had already experienced whatever it was they were spelling, reading, writing, or counting about. That wasn't a good attitude to have but it went unnoticed for the most part until high school.

I was too small to be much of a bully, but if anyone, at any time, wanted to challenge me about what I thought was right, look out. I was truly a stand-up-type kid. But I failed to recognize or read the price tags for my behavior until I joined the marines in 1958.

School had become a real embarrassment for me in many ways. I was always starting but never finishing. By the time I made it to the Dade County School System in 1954, I just wanted to forget about it. Give me a shovel, already. I'll dig a ditch. I had been playing catch-up for years and I never seemed to get caught up. The faster I went the "behinder" I got, and my attitude suffered greatly. Come to think of it, sitting in my room putting model cars together for hours on end with an open tube of glue four or five inches below my nose most likely didn't help my attitude, either. However, at that time it seemed to me to be a lot more fun building model cars than taxing my imagination with some empirical facts about science and stuff like that. What inhaling all those glue fumes did to me exactly, who knows? My brain may have suffered some damage long before I suffered TBI.

Biscayne Gardens Elementary. 1954, four years before high school. I was a fair-haired child and I never seemed to have any popularity problems at all. I was even voted king of my fourth grade class. We had a dance and a crowning ceremony. I was fine until I figured out how far behind I actually was.

My fourth grade teacher, Mr. Bradley, gave me a note one afternoon and instructed me to take it home and read it to my mother. I'll never forget what he had written. The note began,

"Dear Joey" (I hated that name, Joey).

"Never have I seen such enthusiasm for the game of baseball in such a small blond boy. Keep it up. Only, spare a little time for the classroom along the way. It will pay you big dividends one day when you're in the big leagues.

Your friend and teacher,

Mr. Bradley."

How I ever managed to pass the fourth grade is beyond me.

Junior high was another lost cause. The school building was new in 1956. I was in the first class ever to go to North Miami Junior High School. Right off the bat, my homeroom teacher wanted to have a meeting with my parents. Apparently the lady realized how far behind I actually was. I took a note home to my mother at my teacher's request. My mother became very angry after reading it and I recall her saying, among other things,

"What do these people think we're paying them for, anyway?" My mother never did go to see that teacher. Instead she wrote a note and talked to her on the phone. How or what was resolved I never knew.

More bad news in the sixth grade. For the first time in my life I had a physical education teacher that I could not stand. He was overweight and out of shape. He did not like me and I did not like him. He had this rude, somewhat arrogant manner of communicating. In the first field-house meeting, the big idiot made it crystal clear that the only way to get an A in his class was if he liked you or if your father could kick his butt. Well, in the seventh grade I got him again and although we continued our dislike of one another, I did go to see him just to make sure that he knew that although I didn't have a father, I did have a six-foot-four stepfather whose weight I inflated a bit just for the effect. Less than a week later I was on the school track team. Fortunately for me, he found it hard to argue with the stopwatch of another coach. After I made it across the street to high school in 1957, I was told he had gotten himself fired.

Some years later I was looking through a 1957 North Miami Junior High School yearbook. What I found was hard for me to believe. I had been voted one of the ten students most likely to succeed that year. I'm sure that yearbook thing was someone's idea of a joke. I never did find out who put that in there.

By high school I already had many resources to draw from in any given situation. Street smart is what it's called today. The USMC took care of any discipline deficit I may have had by the time I reached the age of twenty-one, but as a young teen I had this strange, nagging desire to belong to someone or something that would demand my loyalty and extreme devotion. Without that, I was simply one more rebellious teenager. I had always felt a real closeness to my mother—at least until she remarried in

1955 and gave birth to my half sister Karen in 1956. Oddly enough given my last statement, I have always felt a real closeness to my half sister—mutual admiration at its best!

On the other hand, I considered her father, in all honesty and in many ways, to be a very strange man. I was not alone. Most of the people in our neighborhood seemed to think of him in that way. I suppose he had his reasons for his ways and perhaps justifiably so. I know I never really figured him out, that's for sure. (I guess you could say with some degree of accuracy that I was a strange kid myself back then—a real free spirit. You might even say that of me today.) I can't say that I knew the man very well at all. I don't think many people did. He was an extra-tall person—six-foot-four at least. He had the largest hands of anyone I had ever met. I often thought about those huge hands and the grip I was sure I could get on a baseball if I had them. Unfortunately the man had absolutely zero interest in athletics. I believe he may have brought some strange ideas home with him from India, where he had been stationed during the Second World War. I know he brought malaria back with him, but when my mother met him in 1954, it was under control. He told me once that quinine worked wonders for him. I don't know. Like I said, I never knew him very well.

Anyhow, I had simply lost my interest in the classroom long before I entered high school, which I did in 1957. I remember one other incident that occurred while I was a freshman at North Miami High School. I was in Spanish class and the teacher asked me to count to ten—in Spanish, of course. Well, after standing and groping for a moment or two, never taking my eyes off my feet, I told her in a very loud and confident tone of voice that all I would ever have to know would be how to count to three in English: "One, two, three, you're out." Her reply came quickly, above the laughter of my classmates: "Uno, dos, tres, and you're out of here."

My love for the game and my ability to play the game only grew stronger as time passed. I had been told on more than one occasion that the scouts were watching. My mother was of the opinion that baseball was a waste of time. I should have bigger and much better fish to fry at the age of fifteen. Come on, Mom, give me a break! (I'm sure I had many unspoken thoughts like that at the time, but I simply didn't talk to my mother or my stepfather like that back then. I can't say I knew anyone who did.)

I often think about the eight ball my mother talked about being born behind. I think I understand and respect what she was saying now but at the time, no way. I also think that the same eight ball my mother blamed for holding her back in her life was in some way hindering her ability to see, exactly, where I was in mine at any given time. Respect is definitely a two-way street.

There were times, many times, when I really felt as though I were not a part of anyone's family at all. It always seemed to me, however, that I simply could not hang on to those feelings or thoughts long enough to do anything that might help change the situation. I guess I had my own agenda, and had had it since my orphanage years. I was very sure that I knew exactly where I was headed with my life. Three strikes and you're out!

Anyway, it seems to me that the only time my folks ever showed much respect or enthusiasm for my love of the game of baseball was when I was working as an umpire for the city of North Miami Beach at age sixteen, and getting paid for it, at that! Actually, I did a good bit of "umping" at age fifteen also. My parents always approved of my making money.

At team functions when parents were invited, I was always the kid whose parents never showed up. The thing that made it even worse, I guess, was the fact that my teammates usually voted me captain of whatever team I happened to be on at the time. (I really don't like sounding like a braggart. I'm simply telling you like it was.)

I believe I would be a bit remiss if I didn't say something about parental involvement here, so I will. Get involved. Now! It just might be too late in the morning. Parental involvement was seriously missing in my life.

Every time I notice the plaques hanging on the wall in our little home office, plaques presented to both my wife and me for school volunteer work, I feel good inside…warm and fuzzy! But I can't help feeling a bit sad for my mother. I try not to disregard the era in which she lived. In contrast, most of the advances that have been made in education have been right on the money. Parental involvement—don't let your kids leave home without it.

Now, a boy without parental involvement living in NMB and going to school in North Miami didn't stand much of a chance of playing high school baseball or any other varsity sport, especially when his grades are poor at best, and mine were indeed poor at their very best—very close to being the worst they could possibly be. The only exceptions were my grades in physical education, which were straight A's at all times (except for sixth grade). Year in and year out, I was always at the top of my class in PE, no matter where I was going to school.

At the request of my freshman year physical education coach, I decided to try out for the high school baseball team. I was hesitant. My grades were really poor, and transportation was a big problem. I honestly believed that if I could just get some help at home I would be okay. The truth is, any help from home at that time probably would have been too little, too late.

I finally made my mind up to do it. I would just have to walk home every day for a couple of weeks. That wouldn't be so bad. The walk was just a little over four miles. If I took the shortest route, cutting through front and back yards along the way, I would make record time. I never walked anywhere anyway. I was always running.

I was a bright and fairly good-looking young man. I was extremely athletic and active. I thought I had a very bright future ahead of me. How should we measure success? I have come to realize that the simple accomplishment of putting on our own shoes each morning is truly a measure of success. If my bell had never been severely rung, would I have been a successful person? Can anyone answer that question? Probably not. Of course, I'm not really sure exactly how far my love for the game of baseball may have taken me, although I do remember what it felt like to put my own spikes on and run like the wind. This much I am certain of: Just like Satchel Paige, I would have still been throwing a baseball at the age of 62. I would never have quit playing baseball if not for all my physical complications. The feeling I get when I sit in a dugout or walk out onto a baseball field even today is far from normal.

At the same time, since I was not producing in the classroom at the level I should have been, a label was sticking to me like epoxy, especially in the mind of my stepfather. That label and buzz word of the 1950s was juvenile delinquent. Many young people, some justly so and some unjustly so, wore that label back then.

I guess the straw that broke the camel's back as far as I was concerned was when, after tryouts had ended and just about a week before the final cut, some members of the school team came into my stepfather's store and requested a donation. (My stepfather had an art store on 125th Street in North Miami.) In no uncertain terms he told those boys that he was of the opinion that his stepson was not worth helping. He simply was not about to give them a donation just so I could play high school baseball. Needless to say, my stepfather and I never hit it off very well. As far as he was concerned, I was a juvenile delinquent and that was that.

Of course, I knew I wasn't a juvenile delinquent. I really wasn't even a bad kid, but an angel I was definitely not. In the eyes of most adults back then, kids were darling little angels when they were sent off to live in orphan homes, but they weren't when they got out. I had been told on occasion that I had all of the ear-marks of a real hood. But I knew that I never wanted to harm anyone, and above all I wanted to do the right thing.

I had been taught right from wrong by some very intelligent people, especially during the time I spent in the Lake Bluff Orphanage. Most of the counselors or dorm parents that I came into contact with during my stay at Lake Bluff Orphanage were professionals. If not, they were students studying at Northwestern University in hopes of becoming professionals.

I was also bright enough by the time I found myself living at home once more to see through an adult of less sincerity and less intelligence than I was used to dealing with. In my case that may not have been the best thing. I recall hearing a small group of adults talking out on the back porch of our home in North Miami Beach. I overheard one of these adults saying, "Joe can really get someone's number in one big hurry." I never did find out what that conversation was all about, but I know one thing for sure: I felt a lot of resentment coming from many adults during my mid teens.

Perhaps the resentment I felt had a lot to do with the fact that I really did have their numbers. But simply being able to see through all of the phony adults in one's life does not necessarily lead one to delinquency. However, it sure can get you in a bunch of trouble, especially when you just can't seem to keep your mouth shut. Most people I knew, both adults and other kids, would tell you that I had a problem in that area. Whatever I was thinking at any given time was more than likely what I was going to say. Smart, fast answers were never a problem for me. This did not always prove to be advantageous when it came to influencing other people or making friends.

I don't think I can tell you for sure why it was that I always seemed to be making friends with people who were called bad seeds and the like, but that's what was happening. If only I had been productive in the class-room, things would have been a lot different. Back in the late 1950s drugs and guns were not much of a problem in North Miami High School. On the other hand, under aged drinking, teen sex and some criminal behavior such as shoplifting, stealing cars, vandalism and criminal mischief seemed to be accelerating, and this type of activity in most cases led to hard core criminal behavior later on down the line. As far as I was concerned the handwriting was on the wall, but I didn't know what to do about much of anything at the time. My life was not moving in the right direction—I did know that. Most of my friends were bad seeds. They were the real juvenile delinquents, and most of them were bound to become losers sooner or later. That great old worn-out idea that you are the company you keep is very hard to find fault with. My new label among my peers was Little Bad Ass. I was becoming a real loser, and was definitely on a fast track to nowhere.

In 1958, after Christmas break, I felt I had to do something drastic in hopes of turning my life around. My chosen course of action was a warped one indeed. I made a conscious decision to do something that would get everyone's attention, including that of a little blond girl who I had an unrelenting crush on. I drove my 1949 Hot Rod Ford at top speed through the school bus loading zone. I often wish I had never done that. The little blond showed little sympathy, if any at all. She asked me if I had lost my mind. I really felt like I didn't have anything left to live for.

Not to worry. I soon remembered that feeling sorry for myself was bad news to say the least. We might all be better off if we could hang on to that thought throughout our lives. After a conference with the school's dean, I figured I could either quit high school and join the service or eventually be expelled. So even though I was certainly not the sharpest knife in the kitchen, this was, as they say, a no-brainer!

CHAPTER 4

I Got Nothing to Lose!

USMC, here I come. Within ninety days of the donation request and the denial thereof, I quit school and joined the marines. (Like I said, I was always running.) Of course, my parents had to sign for me to go into the service at that time (underage, you know), but there really wasn't any hesitation on their part. Not one bit. Uncle Sam wants who? For me it was quit high school and go into the service or…

I remember thinking at that time about one of the counselors I had had while at Lake Bluff. (He is another one of those special people who seems to have found it impossible to completely get lost in the tangled depths of my off again on again memory.) This particular fellow was studying at Northwestern University in hopes of one day becoming a Catholic priest. Mr. Ryan was a tall, thin man who certainly did not need to wear a white hat in order for folks to know he was one of the good guys. He always wore glasses similar to those that were worn years later by the famed rock and roll personality Buddy Holly. The heavy black frames of his glasses made him look as though he had read every book that had ever been written. Everyone liked Mr. Ryan. At first glance he appeared to be a bookworm and perhaps a bit of a wimp, but this first impression soon gave way to one of a magnificent-spirited father figure. This man would read to us almost every night before bedtime. His reading of the *Call of the Wild* by Jack London was terrific.

But it was another story that Mr. Ryan told us that would, in some strange way, influence my decision as to which branch of service I would ultimately join. The counselor told us in a

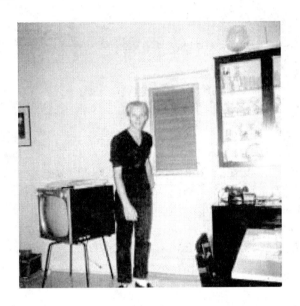

6 weeks before Parris Island

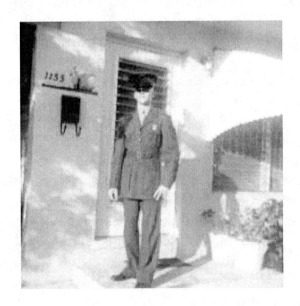

90 Days After Parris Island

cracking voice, as he pulled off his glasses to wipe a tear from his eye, about his older brother and how he had joined the Marine Corps only to lose his life on the beach of some South Pacific island that had been overrun by the Japanese Empire. Mr. Ryan had never forgiven the USMC, and he felt as though they had let his brother down. He had gone on to tell us in no uncertain terms that if we ever had to go into the service for the defense of our country, the Marine Corps should be our very last choice.

Well, after mulling his message over in my mind for a short time, I felt very confident in my rebellious thoughts that the United States Marine Corps may well be my last choice. Possibly the last choice I would ever make. So what? I was rebelling against God and life in general. I perceived my life to be all messed up at best—nothing to lose! Mr. Ryan was fine person whose brother had died for this country of ours, and if that was good enough for Mr. Ryan's brother, it would be good enough for me. It was my country too. The hows, whys and wherefores of Mr. Ryan's advice fell on deaf ears. After all, it was peace-time and the odds might just be in my favor. I don't believe I ever had a real death wish, but my youthful rebellion clearly did not know logic, and four very long years of being at the extreme ready would follow.

Now that I'm well past my youthful rebellion, there are times when I really do try to find some logic in war. The Ryan brothers, war and logic, now that's enough to give most folks a headache, for sure! Me included. But I have very few regrets, if any at all, for having joined the marines. After all, I came home alive. Many other young men did not.

I did have a small problem getting into the USMC in the first place, however. At the ripe old age of seventeen it seemed that my disdain for food in general (the exception being junk food, of course) was becoming evident. It's hard to understand exactly why, but real food like milk, eggs, meat, vegetables, and most anything not fried or with low sugar content was not going to be eaten by me. Orphanage food was the pits, and as for all of the other people who had cooked for me and made me eat (mainly because of all of the other kids who were starving all over the world, or so they said), their food simply did not appeal to me either. Father chef and mother waitress equaled good food in my young mind.

The results of my poor eating habits were a problem when I tried to join the marines in 1958. My 57-inch-tall frame, although extremely wiry and strong for both age and size, was carrying less than 100 pounds of body weight on that glorious day of truancy from NMHS when I became convinced that I was definitely USMC material. Not getting into the United States Marine Corps was out of the question as far as I was concerned.

For me to gain something like 4 pounds in two weeks was not going to be a big problem. My weight fluctuated between 100 pounds and 112 pounds regularly anyway. Every single one of my high school friends was very supportive and helpful with their instruction and advice. One of my best and brightest pals said that what he would do would be to get four pounds of lead fishing sinkers and swallow each one of them. One of the other guys who was standing around while these heartfelt instructions were coming down slapped his hands together in agreement and shouted, "Yeah, and wash them all down with a six-pack!" One of the girls said, "No, that could make him sick or even dead." I replied quickly, "Right. Lead poisoning."

One crazy idea led to another until finally I found myself eating bananas one after another on the day before my final trip down town to see the recruiter. When I told him about the bananas he smiled from ear to ear and said, "Them bananas do it every darn time." My friends and I had all agreed that the banana thing was the best thing to do. And it may have been, at that. My stomach looked and felt a lot heavier, and everyone said they were positive that I had gained the required pounds. Apparently not one of us had the bright idea to put me on a scale before I went back downtown. I had no idea what I now weighed when I talked to the marines in the post office in downtown Miami.

No problem! "110 pounds, right on the money," the USMC recruiter said as he slapped my back. "You're on your way!"

After getting back into the car that was being driven by my best and brightest high school friend, we proceeded to remove the extra weight that we had taped to my ankles and stuffed into my pockets. The recruiter had said 110 pounds, right on the money. Can you believe that? Yes sir, bananas do it every time. I'm positively sure there wasn't any need for the extra weight that day. That salty old buck sergeant never even had me get on a scale.

I couldn't get over the excitement and anticipation that was caused by what I believed the Marine Corps recruiter had told me. There's a lot of truth to the saying that people only hear what they want to hear, especially seventeen-year-old people without very much going for them. Going to Paris for boot camp was almost too much for me to cope with! Somehow, and I guess it's not too surprising given the fact that I had gotten straight F's in geography for some time, I failed to realize that Parris Island was located in South Carolina and definitely not in France.

Talk about a rude awakening when I was given a train ticket to Jacksonville, Florida and a Greyhound Bus ticket from Jacksonville to Yamasee, South Carolina. On the bus ride from Jacksonville to Parris Island, I could not stop thinking about life in Our Good Old LBO. I was trying desperately to convince myself that being in the Marine Corps was going to be something like being a member of Wadsworth 1 (with the potential for a real war added on, of course).

Forget that. Not even close! The only thing the two had in common as far as I could tell was that they both had multiple urinals in what the drill instructors called "the head," and what I had always been told to call "the bathroom."

I stepped off the bus at Parris Island to the tune of "Be Kind to Your Web-footed Friends" by John Philip Sousa. The USMC band was practicing off in the distance. Then, when I heard the guy wearing the far-out hat tell me, among other things, that from now on he was mommy and daddy...it was not a good feeling. We were going to do things his way, no questions asked. I had no idea what I was in for. Changed, transformed, I was. Parris Island was an instant involuntary attitude adjustment for me, for sure. From that point on, I knew I was in some deep stuff. I was about to be changed forever. Even if I had, like a psychologist once told me, quit school and left home to spite my parents, the hurt was on me.

The DIs were moving around rapidly, with uncanny precision, hollering commands like you would not believe, in my face one minute, ten feet away the next. The names I was called on that first day of boot camp in July of 1958 I had never heard before in my entire life, and I was a kid who had played the game many times.

On that day, my first at PI, I was called "Whale Shit." The friendly DI, whose nose was located squarely between my eyes, explained that whale shit is found on the bottom of the ocean. He went on in an extra-loud tone of voice to assure me that I couldn't get much lower than that. (He really needed a breath mint, but you can bet that I was not about to suggest it.) He also called me "Scum of the Earth," "Turd," "Piss Ant," and I can't leave out "Maggot" and "Sack of Shit." He said I was a blond-headed Elvis and told me in no uncertain terms that my ass was grass and he was the lawn mower. After that first day, believe me, it only got worse.

I was shocked again, in a slightly different way, when I caught a glimpse of what looked to me to be a never-ending sea of bald heads moving in unison, with a crimson and gold guide on banner flying in the breeze, moving across what the U.S. Marines call "the grinder." The drill field is what it's called by normal people. It was an incredibly humbling sight indeed for a self-centered, wide-eyed teenage kid. My pneumatic ego went a bit flat. Who am I, Lord, that thou art mindful of me?

I had no idea at all that there would be a physical exam just hours before I was to be officially sworn in to the Marine Corps. I did pass it, though. My weight was not mentioned, and this time more than one person had definitely read the scale that I was told to stand on. A couple hours later the swearing-in ceremony took place. I became a United States Marine eight days after my seventeenth birthday.

Now that you have no doubt caught on to my style of writing, you're probably expecting some funny stories about USMC boot camp, but let me assure you of this: There is absolutely nothing amusing about it. I don't mean to sound like a wise guy, but the whole point of boot camp is to discipline one's thinking. I don't think I laughed at all while there. If I did laugh it was never out loud. Many times I would hear (definitely not see, but hear only. An outstanding maggot's eyes are straight ahead at all times.) some commotion in the ranks as we were standing at attention in formation. A couple of times it was caused by a fellow boot who apparently had made that mistake or a similar one. This always resulted in the DIs doing what they called a bit of thumping. Thumping was for a man's own good, of course! Thump! Thump! That was enough for me. I didn't talk to anyone for ninety days except when answering a drill instructor. "Yes, sir!" or "No, sir!" That's exactly how it was.

One time, a poor guy put his bayonet on his rifle prematurely. No order had been given to do so. If anyone had given the order to fix bayonets everyone had missed it but that string-bean kid from West Virginia. It was stuck! He was stuck! He had absolutely no idea how to get it off. The DI's thought that was hilarious. Here was this seventeen-year-old marine recruit at fixed bayonets, standing at attention in formation, trembling, shaking, out of his mind with anticipation. Yes, sir, for sure. Boots with amusing stories? Not many! Thump! Thump! Thump!

Upon graduating from Parris Island, and in accordance with all USMC rules and regulations, every recruit in Platoon 309, Third Battalion had become a man. Each one of us had completed three months of intensive recruit training. We all had reached a goal that had often seemed unattainable. The hardships and discomforts we all learned to deal with successfully had truly been unspeakable. At this point, as we stood motionless and at attention waiting for the company commander to give the order "Prepare for graduation," every man knew he would proudly wear the name marine for the rest of his natural life. The order was given and anticipation made its way through the ranks. We all knew that that order would soon be followed by another order.

Our drill instructor finally gave that order. It was the order to dismiss that every last one of us had been waiting to carry out since we arrived at PI. The DI dismissed his platoon of dedicated marines, Platoon 309, for the last time. He was both proud and confident of the fact that he had transformed boys into men and men into marines.

Our new title had not been earned easily. Although each man was extremely proud and extremely happy that our recruit training had finally come to an end, the degree of discipline we had all been subjected to and had attained was indelible. As we moved slowly toward the waiting buses—buses that would take us to Camp Lejuine, North Carolina for advanced infantry training, our silence was without question a golden silence.

During our trip to Camp Lejuine, if there was any laughter or talking at all it remained extremely reserved. Transformed! Indeed we had been. I know that I had tried very hard for the past three months to convince myself to forget how to talk completely. Listening had become far more important to me. Each one of us had learned how to listen and how to get in touch with ourselves in a way that was truly and uniquely beneficial to the individual marine when faced with adversity of any kind. Now, both jointly and severally, the application of our boot camp training at PI would be put to the test.

To a man, not one of us had any real idea what life would be like for us during the next twelve weeks of advanced infantry training. One thing we all seemed to have more than a little notion of, however, was that we were all bound to be snooping and pooping deep in the woods of North Carolina for some time. In very short order we were going to gain even more of an understanding of the importance of a marine platoon to function as one man. What to do with a bayonet and how to do it would be learned by every man, even the string-bean from West by God. Personally, I never knew how close I could get to another man until we all spent a few nights in below freezing temperatures. Body heat can keep a couple of extra-lean seventeen-year-old marines from freezing their butts off.

And orders that are carried out sharply, precisely, and confidently will, for the most part, keep you from getting your butt *shot* off. But even if things didn't always work out exactly as planned, the idea was to carry on the age-old Marine Corps legacy.

They died with their boots on, fought like hell and took with them every bastard they possibly could. I never saw any combat myself (close, but no cigar), but at the ready I was at all times. I thank God that I never had to kill or be killed or stand by while another human being was butchered in my sight.

I do know this for certain: I will, until the day I die, tell anyone at any time and without any reservation just how much we all owe to those men and women who have served in any branch of the service in the defense of the United States of America. I am extraordinarily proud to know anyone who truly bleeds red, white, and blue.

Anyhow, the notions we all had about Marine Corps life and our infantry training at Lejuine were mostly right on. We were convinced that our infantry training would go on for an eternity or perhaps until General George Custer of the Seventh Calvary, United States Army was resurrected and given command of the USMC, whichever came first. Neither solution seemed to be forthcoming. All of us, to a man, were definitely ready to snoop and poop in the woods forever at the wish of any USMC officer, whoever he might be.

Then, just as suddenly as we found ourselves in the woods, we were out of the woods. I mean completely out of the woods, both mentally and physically. It was almost as though we had never been subjected to any of it at all. The advanced infantry training had been completed. Every man knew how to do it and was confident in his ability to do it. Lean, mean, fighting machines we had all become.

"Blakemore, Benzenhofer, and Blankenship, get up here!" That was the order that reverberated throughout our barracks on the morning we three boots (a "boot" in the corps is a marine fresh out of boot camp) were given our first duty assignments. "You three lucky maggots are shipping out to the Second Marine Air Wing just down the road at Cherry Point." We were told by some fancy-looking corporal wearing bloused and brightly gleaming spit-shined boots. The immaculate corporal also ordered us to get our gear and report to the sergeant holding the clipboard who was standing next to the PC (personnel carrier) parked directly in front of our barracks. "Yes, sir!" was our only reply.

The marine with a worn-out-looking clipboard was an older logistics sergeant with a couple of combat and occupational ribbons on his chest and a look of stone on his face. His eyes met mine and I tried very hard to give him back the same look of emptiness that I saw. A faint smile followed and he spoke. "Okay, 'Youngblood', these are your papers. Don't lose the damn things." "Yes, sir!" I replied as sharply as I could. (The three of us, like all boots, would be calling every PFC or better "sir" for some time to come! Shoot! I'm still in the habit of calling most everyone sir and I've been out of the corps for many years.) I felt his gaze fall from mine as he handed my two new buddies their papers. He then turned toward a PFC who was the apparent driver of the PC and said, "Mount up."

We all quickly climbed into the back of that old WWII PC. Just like that logistics sergeant, I'm sure that old truck had more time in the chow line than the three of us had in the corps.

The three of us had been given the MOS (Military Occupational Specialty) of 3500—that of a Marine Corps driver. Although we had never seen one another before that morning (we had all come from different platoons at PI), there was that instant USMC camaraderie. We knew we were going to be together for a while and we knew also, beyond any doubt, that we could depend on each other without question. At the same time, the phrase 'here today and gone tomorrow' was never far from our thoughts. That shot of transformation we had been given at PI was some powerful stuff ... really!

'Just down the road' turned out to be about 250 miles. It seems to me that the very next day we were learning to drive big trucks, stay awake and alert all night, be a designated driver, and refuel all emergency cradsh crew vehicles brought over to us from the flight line throughout the night.

"We got 'two bys,' 'four bys,' 'six bys,' and those big MFs that bend in the middle and say 'shh- shh.' You call, we haul you all. If we can't truck it, &#%@ it!" That would become our slogan for the next three and a half years. (I for one could still taste the soap that my mother had used when she washed out my filthy little mouth for saying something a lot nicer than that. As a matter of fact, had she known, my mother would have gone through a couple dozen bars of soap per day for the next forty-two months, no doubt.)

The oldest member of our newly formed little threesome seemed to be very amused with the name of our new duty station. "Cherry Point. Do you get it?" he asked a couple of times. "Yeah! I get it!" I finally shouted in my very best all-knowing and all-understanding, extremely mature-sounding tone of voice. I really didn't. And at the same time I really didn't think he knew all that much either.

I remember one night in particular when I had sentry and gasman duty. I had only been at Cherry Point for about two weeks. It was one of those freezing North Carolina nights. There had to be a foot of snow on the ground and a light flurry still falling. The duty of the sentry and gasman is to serve as a type of fire watch and refuel the emergency vehicles of the various crash crews in the area. He is also at all times to be prepared to carry out orders he is given by the night dispatcher.

This particular night dispatcher was an old busted-down PFC who seemed to very much enjoy ordering me around while at the same time referring to me as Short Round or Youngblood. I must admit I kind of liked being around this old salt myself.

At about 3:30 in the morning on this particular cold and snowy night, Pappy, as the other marines called him, sent me off into the night to check all of the doors in the immediate area. I was to try each one to make certain that all were secured. After about 30 minutes of stomping around in the snow and making sure that the area was definitely secure, I returned to the outside dispatcher window with my report. Pappy told me that I had done an outstanding job and that he wanted me to go get the mule and pull one of the school buses off the ready line. Two other marines, I was told, were having a very hard time getting bus number 42 to start, and it had to make an early morning school run to a school some thirty-five miles away.

Well, I had never before seen the mule and had absolutely no idea where to look for it, but I figured it was far better for me to take off looking for that mule than it would be for me to try and explain my ignorance of something like that to Pappy. About fifteen minutes later I returned to the dispatch window, peered inside and stated in that all-confident, extra-mature tone of voice that I mentioned earlier, "I can't even find his stall!" Every man within earshot was laughing and the night dispatcher shook his head and called me a shitbird.

I really made some good friends that night, and more than one person went out of his way to explain that the mule was actually a piece of US Navy equipment usually used for pushing vehicles and not for pulling them. Just to be on the safe side and to make certain they had made their point, some added, "You don't feed the mule corn and it hasn't got a stall." I was told later that the whole mule thing was one of the night dispatcher's ways of having fun with the new boots.

Approximately forty-five minutes after the sun had come up and established a new day, all the night duty personnel were dismissed. Still feeling somewhat embarrassed over falling for the old mule gag, I headed off alone through the lightly falling snow toward the barracks that I had previously been assigned to. Both Blankenship and Benzenhofer passed by me as they were headed toward the motor pool to report for duty that morning. As they were passing me by, I heard Benzenhofer say, "Hey Blakemore, did you ever find that mule?" My reply was quick. "Hell yes! If you two shitbirds would have been looking for it, you would still be out there." I think it was the new addition to my vocabulary that really cracked them both up more than anything else.

Adjusting to duty at Cherry Point was not that bad, and very soon all three of us were performing our duties in a confident and responsible manner. Soon we were driving everything from staff cars to dump trucks to school busses, not to mention those two bys, four bys, and six bys that I spoke of earlier.

Of course, we were constantly reminded that every enlisted man in the Marine Corps was a basic rifleman. The Marine Corps, at that time, made sure that every enlisted marine qualified yearly with the M1 rifle. (I had just barely managed to qualify at Parris Island due to the confusion of the recruit next to me. He had managed to inadvertently fire on my target in the middle of a South Carolina summer rain storm.)

Within the first six months of being stationed at Cherry Point I found myself headed off to the rifle range again. Trying to convince myself that I would do much better this time than I had done the time before was not easy, but ultimately I was able to do it. As a matter of fact, I shot expertly that year, and every year after that for the remainder of my four-year enlistment. I was very proud of my marksmanship accomplishments and I let all of my superiors know that I wanted to go to sniper school.

It was an incident with a school bus a little bit later on that would ultimately point me in the direction of school.

Unfortunately, or perhaps fortunately, depending upon your point of view, sniper school was not the kind of school that the Marine Corps had in mind for me.

On my very first school bus run, a small group of parents who were apparently concerned about my extremely youthful appearance called my commanding officer, the CO of my motor transport outfit at Cherry Point. The commanding officer was informed that these folks thought that one of the school kids had taken off with a school bus. Although I was just about to turn eighteen years old at the time, I could very easily have passed for a fourteen-year-old.

One day soon after that I was standing in the chow line at the mess hall with a few other guys from the motor pool when the same old night dispatcher, Pappy, said, "That's a real bitch. You're old enough to be a marine, but Youngblood, you're much too young-looking to die."

Most of us had learned to take whatever the old man said with a grain of salt. Pappy was a forty-six-year-old PFC who had seen it all. He had been busted many times and he liked to tell anyone who would listen that the first time he was busted was for having buffalo shit on his bow and arrow. It seems to me, though, that it was the following day that I got the news from my CO that my orders were being cut—orders that would send me to a place called Montford Point for six weeks of intense automotive mechanic training.

Upon graduating from the Marine Corps School of Advanced Automotive Mechanic Training, most marines swear that they can disassemble a Jeep engine and reassemble it blindfolded. Believe me, some of us could, and in short order at that! We had all earned a new MOS as well. Our new MOS was 3516—we were all United States Marine Corps mechanics. I was soon to be elevated in rank to PFC (private first class) and sent back to the motor pool at Cherry Point, North Carolina.

Upon my arrival back at my former duty station, I received my first stripe, a United States Safe Driving Award, and I was told that I had an unlimited military driver's license. After having been in the Marine Corps for less than 2 years, I had become the only automotive mechanic stationed at Cherry Point, Second Marine Air Wing, USMC.

At that time I still didn't appear to be as old as I was, and I was not all that old anyway. Like I said, I was proud! I was extraordinarily proud! However, proud is probably not the most descriptive word we could use here. Cocky is a better word by far, and believe me I know.

"Blakemore, you have really got it made!" That was what everyone was thinking and that was what everyone was saying. Yes! I really did believe that I had it made, and for life at that.

I was no longer working with the other people in the motor pool. Blankenship was still a driver and Benzenhofer had been kicked out of the marines for having lied about his age in order to get in in the first place. Poor guy. It seems that although Ben certainly was a lot older-looking than I was, he was actually sixteen months or so my junior. We all hated to see him go. He really was one hell of a marine. He made a great drinking buddy and he always told us stories about how he loved to chase the 'hos' back home in Youngstown, Ohio.

I was no longer a driver, of course, and I had been told to, now get this, report to the Civil Service Heavy Equipment Maintenance Shop located in a very large WWII airplane hangar on the east side of our motor pool compound.

The experience I was gaining was invaluable and I knew it. Officers would bring their lawn mowers to me for repair and I was truly dumbfounded by the respect I was receiving. I loved working with heavy equipment as well. Swinging around in mid air on a crane cable and using a two-pound hammer and a marlin spike to drive large steel pins out of large sections of steel crane boom was fantastic fun.

Everything was going my way. I didn't even have to make our usual early morning formation. I didn't have to wear the uniform of the day. I did, however, have to report for nighttime driver duty once every ten days.

When my name came up for dreaded mess duty—a duty that usually lasted ninety days—I would be driving a deuce and a half (two by) and delivering commissary supplies to all of the mess halls. No one in his right mind wanted to catch mess duty, but if that was the worst job I ever had to do I would remain a happy camper.

Don't get the wrong idea about life in the Marine Corps. It was never easy going. On the contrary, it was at all times tough sledding. Work, work, and more work, and at all times you have got to be ready to move out at a moment's notice. Just where you were bound, or when you might be leaving, you never knew. If you're in the right place at the right time you will be back.

I admit that compared to most other guys in my outfit, I had it made. I believed that I had it made in a couple of different ways. First off, I knew I was a well-trained mechanic and I figured I could do that type of work as a civilian for the rest of my life.

If, on the other hand, my choice was to stay in the corps for life, I was in a specialized field, and making rank would therefore not be a problem. I had become experienced in automotive mechanics and in heavy equipment mechanics as well, and all before my nineteenth birthday. Of course baseball, I was sure, would be in the cards for me sooner or later.

As a matter of fact, the only thing that seemed missing in my life was baseball. I just didn't seem to find any time to play. There were no organized baseball teams at the Point at that time. Strangely enough, I had no sooner mentioned that fact to a few of the marines around the motor pool and to a few of the civil service workers I worked with as well, when a request for ballplayers appeared on the bulletin board in the drivers' ready room. One of the air wing squadrons had decided to organize a baseball team and they were willing to look at anyone who wanted to try out.

Without any problem I was selected, and after a couple of weeks of practice we were ready to play our first game. A group of Marine Corps pilots had gotten the whole thing off the ground in hopes of being able to develop a schedule that would last throughout the entire baseball season. Well, we lost our first game. We really didn't have much in the way of pitching.

All of these young lieutenants and a couple of captains as well (one was the captain of the newly formed team) had been calling me their star utility player from the outset. In our first game I played three different positions, and if the game had not ended when it did I'm sure they would have moved me to the pitcher's mound next.

In the last of the ninth with the tying run on first base, I recorded the last out. I hit a fastball that was just a little bit outside the strike zone deep into right centerfield. The opposition's fleet-footed centerfielder hauled the ball in, making the catch look routine. I was mumbling to myself, saying something about not having gotten enough of it and that I probably should have simply pocked the darn thing for a single, when I realized I was in the presence of what I'd considered to be some very superior humans. (USMC commissioned officers are superior, and as a young marine you never question that.) Two of them wanted to know where I had ever learned to play baseball like that. I was as polite as I could be but more than a little bit intimidated. I simply could not keep from smiling and fidgeting around. Finally I managed to say that I had been playing the game all of my life. I followed that up with, "Thanks a lot, sirs," as I turned and walked off in the direction of my barracks.

I felt a strange sense of embarrassment and at the same time I had enjoyed hearing the things they said. As I walked away I heard one of them say something I would remember later on in Okinawa, halfway around the world: "With an arm like that kid has, he could be pitching in the pros some day." As I headed toward my barracks, my walking soon became jogging and my jogging eventually became a fifty-yard dash. I was trying to slow down enough to open the barracks door and still maintain the momentum needed to fly up the stairs. I had been telling myself while in anticipation of the upcoming stairwell that if those guys could not play ball any better than that, then I could easily learn to fly, and not just up a stairwell, either... I'm talking jets! You can't be thrown in the brig for what you're thinking. Superior humans?

Well, that was our first and last game at the Point. It seems as though this group of superior beings could not get it together. Ego was apparently a big problem for some of them. Unbeknownst to me at the time, the first and last organized baseball game of the 1959 baseball season at Cherry Point would also be the last organized ball game that this kid, this boy of summer, would ever be a part of.

Actually, I experienced life on the high seas before I turned nineteen years old. Like I said before, we never knew where or when we might ship out, and so it was. When you hear that squawk box snap on in the hold of a troop transport ship and the squid on the other end is hollering "General quarters! General quarters!" a chill like you have never experienced before in your young life runs up and down your spine. When the order has not been prefaced by the words, "This is just a drill," a sickening flood of pent-up emotion staggers your very existence.

Once, during some sort of a red alert that caused a bunch of us North Carolina Jarheads to float, at the courtesy of the USN, of course, for a couple of months off the coast of…where, I'm not exactly sure to this day, I suddenly realized that a marine who happened to be a few rungs higher on the stairwell leading topside was losing his breakfast big time. Well, I'm sure you have heard the saying about what always runs downhill. Let me assure you that it was moving rapidly downhill in my direction. To bear the unbearable is to truly understand that death itself is simply part and parcel of living. I could only pray that a good hot shower and a change of utilities would soon be in the offing as opposed to a blood bath on the beach.

My second trip to sea would be a lot tamer, though much longer in duration. I was going to be sent to Okinawa to serve out my last year of military service. I was pleased with that and looked at this move as more of the same. I had it made!

After joining the USMC, my desire to play professional baseball became my covert operation once again. The desire had surfaced for a very short time while I was stationed at Cherry Point, North Carolina, only to be forced back into obscurity when the Cherry Point baseball team was disbanded due to the over-inflated egos of some marines with wings. But I was about to be given the chance I had been waiting for. The last year of my enlistment was spent on the Rock. The Rock is the name the marines have given to the Ryukyuan Island known as Okinawa. I would be given the opportunity to try out for the all-service baseball team there.

My efforts were rewarded, and my thoughts of being extra special when it came to playing baseball were reinforced, when I was selected for that team. I felt as though I had finally made it, big time. I had my ticket in my hand, and I was really on my way. The exposure I would get would be a dream come true.

I guess I forgot all about my indestructible, carefree, don't-give-a-damn attitude toward life, which I figure is more than likely genetic. It was bound to derail my train sooner or later. Sooner it was.

Less than five-days after being selected for the all-service team in Okinawa, I injured my left knee. I had injured it earlier that same year while on some training maneuvers. At that time, a navy corpsman had told me that I had simply sprained my knee. Within a few hours I was walking around, just fine, like nothing had ever happened. Any swelling was quick to subside. I did notice a small puffy spot just below and to the right of my left kneecap, but in about a week it was gone, too, or so I thought. Some three weeks later I had all but forgotten about it.

This time, I was running wind sprints in the outfield when I stepped into this hole that was obviously not supposed to be there. It was not a very deep hole at all, but at that moment I was very much aware of the fact that my new coach was eyeballing my every move, so in an attempt to show off my 4:4 – 4:3 – speed, I was running in the outfield with reckless abandon.

The moment I stepped into that darn hole I knew I was in big trouble. My first reaction was to try not to give in to the excruciating pain. I would fake it and try to look as if I were attempting to walk off a cramp. I managed to get off the field and into a nearby jeep with the help of another player just as the coach called an end to practice.

The minute I got back to my own outfit I requested permission to go to sickbay. I was ordered to report to a navy doctor who told me that my knee was in much worse shape than anyone had ever told me before.

I remember feeling very sick inside, and after a few confirming X-rays I found myself wearing a cast that extended from the back of my butt to my left ankle. The cast was plaster of Paris, not lightweight fiberglass like we have today. No one knew anything at all about arthroscopic surgery, either. No one ever referred to my problem as a meniscus tear. The terminology that was used back then was simply "torn cartilage of the left knee." It really didn't matter what they called it. There wasn't anything that the best of orthopedic surgeons could do to repair such an injury back then. I was definitely too early and more than one dollar too short.

Well, as I've already told you, I felt very sick inside, indeed, wearing my newly formed bright white cast. Having to hop and swinging my left leg in order to get around on my new crutches was not my cup of tea. Needless to say this did not make me a very happy camper at all!

Once I got back to our Quonset hut at Camp Hague, my buddies started calling me "Chester", like the guy on the TV program "Gunsmoke". I remember thinking at that time, "They all should be calling me Matt, not Chester. After all, Matt had blazing speed…"

Anyway, with my discharge date less than one year away, I was rapidly becoming a short-timer. There wasn't any way for me to pick up my transfer from H. Q. and follow through with the move to special services. My knee simply was not going to heal that quickly. Of course I didn't know it at the time, but my knee wasn't ever going to heal.

One thing I knew for sure: I would not be added to the roster in that condition. I knew there was definitely no chance at all for me to fake it, either. I could all but feel that short-timer's stick in my hand. (A short-timer's stick is a fancy little stick that many marines carry around with them when they are near the end of their enlistment.)

With tear-threatened eyes I reported to the man who was supposed to be my new coach. He was a warrant officer and had been in the corps for most of his life. He was one truly salty individual, for sure. He had also been a student of the game of baseball for many years. I knew beyond a shadow of a doubt that by the time I entered his hatch (that's Marine Corps jargon for door), he was already well aware of what was going on with me. He took one look at me and mumbled in a barely audible tone, "Son of a bitch." I forced a smile and shrugged my already stooped shoulders, while leaning on my new walking apparatus.

"Well, Blakemore, promise me this," he said with a slight smile on his face. "You will never stop playing baseball." My reply was a sharp "Yes, sir!" as I quickly spun around on my crutches and moved out of his sight. Holding the tears back (big boys don't cry), I was all choked up and I never looked back.

I really wanted to keep the promise I had made to that Marine Corps coach even more than my father wanted to keep his big 1937 Indian back in 1944—in other words, one big bunch. I would have loved to be able to play baseball at that level. Gaining that exposure and experience would have been super. I was determined to try my best, but baseball went to the back burner yet again.

While on board the USN transport ship USS Okanogan, coming back across the big pond (that's USMC talk for Pacific Ocean) headed stateside, I skimmed through a book. Some big league pitcher had written it. It was all about some crazy thing called kinesiology. I didn't know anything about that stuff, but the book made a lot of sense to me. Up until my knee problem, I had felt certain that I had what that guy was writing about working within me. I could just feel that energy flow.

I'm not embarrassed to tell you I thought the feeling was spiritual, maybe even supernatural as a matter of fact. I think maybe I had that super feeling for the first time in Okinawa. Or, maybe the first time (I'm not at all sure it was the same thing, though) was way back in Pony League. That time, it seems to me, I hit a ball a good deal farther than my usual distance. And once, in high school, I was playing flag football and had to jump to catch a pass. Well, I jumped all right, and reached as high as I possibly could. I really can't tell you how, but I went up as high as I could go. Then I shot up about four inches higher and caught that ball. The PE coach saw me and shook his head in disbelief. One of the other boys asked me how in the hell I did that. I remember pointing to the sky, shaking my head, and walking off.

Anyway, I knew I had felt something good. It was a great feeling, real smooth, like everything was working together without a hitch. There was more to it than that, though. There had been this, what I called "super energy rush" from my toes to my fingers. It was a feeling that I can only describe as supercharged perfection. No, it didn't happen all the time, but I had always known it was there within my reach.

To tell you the truth, I never felt that feeling again after my knee injury, but I certainly wanted to, for sure. I tried and I tried, but it was gone. Cartilage does not repair itself. At that point, the weak link in my supernatural chain was my left knee, and I had felt that weakness on more than one occasion.

At the age of sixty-one, I still find myself in some kind of a weird daydream at times. I'm playing baseball at Lake Bluff, I'm playing baseball in Miami, and I'm playing baseball in the USMC. In an extremely odd sort of way those dreams always become tangled up with each other and mingle with other things that I can't seem to make out clearly. My baseball dreams always appear to come to an end in my stepfather's art store with me waving goodbye from the fan tail of a troop transport ship headed off to Paris, France. Very strange!

My entire Marine Corps experience was an eye-opener to say the least. The USMC is not for everyone. Perhaps, it's not for anyone. But in the words of Bobby Dylan, "When you got nothing, you got nothing to lose."

I am very proud to have been a United States Marine and I am prouder still of what the USMC has meant to this country of ours. They boldly spilled a lot of blood for the sake of peace and freedom for all, and many of them are no longer standing. God bless them all, the long, the short and the tall!

By the end of my four-year enlistment, I was a very mature, very proud, extremely gung ho young man of twenty-one. I had become accustomed to things running in a smooth and orderly fashion.

I had considered the marines a good career to have, and if I had not screwed up my knee I'm sure I would have re-enlisted. Uncle Sam had offered me a decent deal to do so. But with my knee the way it was and my baseball ideas the way they were, I figured my best shot was as a civilian. So one, two, three, I'm out of there.

CHAPTER 5

Back Home Again?

Ninety days later I was out of my cast. Thirty days after that I was out of the Marine Corps with an honorable discharge. I was asked at that time to sign some sort of a medical release form pertaining to my knee injury, so I felt relatively sure that I would never be asked to serve another day of active military service again in my lifetime.

With Vietnam getting hotter every day, I did have some mixed emotions about that. After all, the only reasons I had for joining the ranks of Uncle Sam's Misguided Children were a real sense of patriotism and a shot at upward mobility—something I was absolutely not getting on the home front. At the very worst, I figured, I would never come home alive. At the very best, I might come home a celebrated hero with a battlefield commission. Of course, if neither one of those things came about, at least, I thought, I was sure to get some good training and education, and the chance to play baseball was always in the back of my mind. In spite of everything, that's exactly what I got: training, education, and the chance to play ball. You might say the USMC had given me a crash course in geography and many other subjects as well. I even got my high school equivalency USFFI-GED during my four-year enlistment. I was well trained in the fields of auto and heavy equipment mechanics.

I was one very proud, bright-eyed, gung ho ex-marine, for sure. I figured I was on my way to the good life, and that the American dream and all that other good stuff were definitely on the horizon. But that's not exactly how things worked out.

My accident, like I said, took place in 1963, but I'm not going there yet. Hang on. I want to tell you a little bit about those early years, the stage-setting years, of my adult life—life before TBI. Again, who a person was before TBI can be extremely important in determining who a person may become after TBI.

I really thought that I had all my bases covered, and all of my little ducklings in a row as well, when it came to having to spend only a short time in my stepfather's home. Total independence for me, and soon: that was my only agenda. Staying with my parents for a couple of weeks looked as though it was the best thing for me to do. They both agreed that it would be okay, and I reassured them that I had everything all figured out.

All of the jobs that were of any interest to me at that time would be found in the south Miami area. My folks and their home were located in northeast Miami. Getting and holding onto a job could be a tough proposition without a dependable set of wheels. Making sure that I had a car was my number one priority.

I was going to buy a used car in San Diego, California with part of the severance pay I had received from the corps. For me to spend money on a bus ticket to Miami was out of the question. It seemed to me to be a waste of both time and money. The right car was all that was needed. And driving cross-country might even be a lot of fun. You know I just had to be thinking of "Route 66", the hot TV show and all that stuff. I did know for certain that once I was back in North Miami Beach, transportation, good dependable transportation, would definitely be the key to my success. Yes sir, a nice used car would do fine. Just so it could get me to Florida and allow me to get around Greater Miami.

I figured that the trip from coast to coast would take no more than four days. Another marine, who had been discharged at the same time that I had, planned to take a bus to his home in Kerrick, Texas. He told me that he lived way up in northern

Texas, almost in southern Oklahoma. Since I was planning to drive through Texas anyway, he had an outstanding opportunity to save himself some money, and he would not be faced with the hassle of getting a ride into downtown San Diego in order to catch a Greyhound bus. He said he hated riding on a bus. So I let him know right off that if he, instead, would give me the cost of his bus ticket less thirty bucks, plus do some of the driving along the way, the trip would be much better for him and for me, too. He thought it was a great idea and assured me that he would be ready to move out when ever I was. (USMC talk for "Lets ride, Clyde.")

The very next morning I got a ride to San Diego and within a couple of hours the bill of sale and the title to the car of my dreams were both in my brand-new genuine leather wallet (hand made in Mexico). This had to be the deal of a lifetime (the car, not the wallet), you bet!

The owners of that car lot saw me, or some other young man with a similar MO, coming their way a long time before I ever got there, I'm sure. Did they ever! Like some people say, anything past the end of my own nose was not being seen clearly at all. A fool and his money are soon parted. Then there's this one: hindsight is always better than foresight! And yet another: Timing is everything! Just why so many of those wise old adages seem to have been afterthoughts for the first twenty some odd years of my life, I'm not at all sure. TBI had not yet befallen me.

The car was an extra-clean-looking 1958 Oldsmobile convertible. Very shiny—glittering, even. That probably had a lot to do with it, for sure! The top had to be moved up and down by hand. The motor had apparently burned up at some point, but that was no big deal. The salesman and I agreed it could be replaced later. The car had four good-looking tires on it and a spare tire in the trunk that looked like it had never been on the ground. All of the tires were recapped, no doubt, but they were sure to keep me rolling around for some time. The big GM engine appeared to be in pretty good shape. It really did! I know I looked it over really well, and I had asked all of the right questions. The radiator didn't show the first sign of ever overheating. It looked really good—not new, of course, but clean.

Thinking back, the entire engine looked super clean—perhaps a bit too clean, at that. Knowing for sure that I could fix any problems on that car by myself and save some big bucks was really limiting my sight to a large degree. The salesman (only after I had pointed it out) did say that the car had a slight oil leak but that he did not think it was a main bearing or anything major like that. Leaking gaskets or seals? Not a biggie, I told myself! This was definitely the car for me! Fixing it? Shoot! Rebuilding it would be no sweat at all. Of course, that San Diego used car salesman and I both agreed that if I were going to drive cross-country I would certainly have to keep my eye on the oil situation. I told the salesman that I could buy a case of motor oil and put it in the trunk before I headed for the East Coast. Then he handed me the keys.

I drove the car around the block, down the street and back. The used Olds ran really well and it drove and handled nicely. It wasn't burning any oil to speak of, and I felt sure of that after taking a good look at the tail pipe. The inside of the tail pipe was a nice pale tan color. Just the color the tail pipe of an automobile should have been before the automotive world was introduced to the catalytic converter in 1975. According to the heat gauge on the dashboard, the big GM V-8 mill was staying really cool. Without too much help from the salesman, I soon became convinced that this car was in good enough condition to travel coast to coast and then some. In less than thirty minutes I drove back onto the used car lot and gave the man $600 in cash. That salesman was a fine guy. He winked and told me to forget about any tax.

I couldn't wait to get it across the United States to Florida, where I could do all the work required to fix it up like new and even better than new. Back in NMB with my own car and a good job…independence at last. Hot dog! Miami, Florida, here I come. Far from being a wet behind the ears seventeen-year-old kid, I had moved headlong into manhood. Miami would be my Big Apple!

Anyway, that very clean canary yellow Oldsmobile convertible was mine and that was one thing I was absolutely sure of. I figured that the trip from coast to coast would take no more than four days. A sucker is born every minute.

Later that same afternoon I returned to the Marine Corps base at San Diego and found the other former marine who would be traveling with me as far as Texas. I had expressed my hopes of traveling Route 66 to him earlier, and while I was off buying my dream car he was doing a little map reading. He informed me that Route 66 was not the route we wanted to travel unless we wanted to wind up in Chicago. If I knew what the future had in store for me, I would have gone straight to Chicago in the first place. Or better yet, I would have never seen the Windy City again in my lifetime. Believe me!

My new number one buddy had our trip all mapped out and was eager to get my approval. I was very happy to find that he had rounded up a couple more people for the trip. One of them was not going very far. He was a marine reservist who had just finished up his first yearly ninety-day commitment, and he needed a lift to his home in Palo Verde, California. Palo Verde was a little bit out of the way, about fifty miles north of where my new map maker had planned for us to enter Nevada, but the idea of putting more money into my new wallet took precedence, and on top of that I really liked the kid. He said he was seventeen but he looked older somehow. Maybe it was his height. He was over six feet, I'm sure. There weren't any stripes on his sleeve, but you got the impression that there should have been and there would be soon. If you can imagine a cross between Gomer Pyle and John Wayne, then you are in the right ballpark when it comes to a visual perception of this particular jarhead. He called everyone sir and I can't tell you that I ever met a more gung ho marine in my life.

The other guy my ex-marine buddy and map-maker extraordinaire had managed to interest in our money-saving venture was going home to New Mexico on a thirty-day leave. This guy had only been in the corps for a couple of years. He was a lance corporal and seemed to have a lot in common with the man who had rounded him up for our trip. Both were of average stature, and were well disciplined recon marines. We were all lance corporals except for good old Gomer Wayne Pyle.

Of course my number one buddy was now an ex-marine. (Everyone called us ex- marines back then, but nowadays we're called former marines. That's because a marine never becomes an ex- marine. Once a marine, always a marine.) Just like me, my number one buddy was proud of his new status.

So that was it. The four of us would be moving out at 0600 hours. Moving out! For two of us it was moving out for the last time. Speaking of time, telling time the military way was no longer necessary, either. Many of those no longer necessary USMC-type things, it seems to me, take forever to get rid of. Anyway, by 0700, the front bumper of my dream car was getting closer to the home of John Gomer Wayne Pyle and Palo Verde, California.

The car radio worked just fine right up until we dropped off our stand-out reservist. The radio suddenly went dead right in the middle of a new hit song by Chubby Checker. I thought it was just a fuse, but that was not the problem. Even to this day, I'm not sure what was wrong with that radio, but when it died you might say the cloud I had been sitting on fell to earth like a rock. Down, I was.

The oil situation was not looking that bad by the time we hit the city limits of Palo Verde, but in reality I had a long, long way to go. A dream car without a radio was for sure not a good thing. I had known many kids in high school who had more of an interest in their car radios than they had in their cars. Keeping my word to that extremely honest, always straight-talking and up-front used car salesman, I had my case of motor oil in my trunk. But motor oil was not a cure for the car radio, nor was it a cure for some of the dashboard and interior lights that refused to come on.

Thoughts of having fouled up big time were being rapidly incorporated into my belief system. Hindsight is what? The silence caused by the radio going south was finally eliminated by the small portable radio of a hitchhiking sailor we stopped to pick up about thirty miles after crossing over into Nevada. (Actually there were three of the navy's proudest on the roadside, but we decided we only had room for one.) The fellow who jumped into the back seat of my sharp-looking Olds convertible said that he did not have much money, but if we could get him to New Orleans he would help buy gas along the way. He handed me his small portable radio and told me to set it on the dash. That sailor boy had picked up very quickly on the fact that our radio was not working.

After checking and adding a quart or more of motor oil, we were rolling down that eastbound highway once again, this time to the sound of "Raindrops" (so many raindrops). We had never once put the convertible top up since leaving California.

Now, very early on our third day and just inside New Mexico, for the first time on our open-air trek we all felt some very real raindrops. My number one good buddy, the other ex-marine in the group, was driving at the time. We all said "Rain!" in unison and he pulled over and stopped the car. Everyone jumped out and helped put the top up. As you know, I knew the convertible top's motor was shot. That stop to put up the top manually resembled a well-planned pit stop during the running of the Indianapolis 500.

Back on the road again in seconds flat, we traveled a mile, or perhaps less than that, to that proverbial gas station in the middle of nowhere. As most young servicemen, ex and former included, we all wanted a cold beer and once again oil was needed in that big V-8 engine. More was needed this time than the time before. At that point I was not feeling as down as I had been feeling a mere forty-eight hours or so ago when the radio died. That Navy man's little sound box had helped a great deal in that regard. Music does that for many of us, I guess. The cold beer did its best as well.

The reading I was getting from my dashboard heat gauge, however, was not at all cool. Wouldn't you just know it? That particular dash light was working well. That had to be a good thing. But would it prove to be of any significance at all? I was determined to fight toward that end. If I could only keep my engine cool!

I told myself to keep on plugging even though my dream appeared to be becoming a nightmare. I fought on through the night, stopping and starting, empty oil can after empty oil can. This was not fun, but after all, there wasn't anyone shooting at us, we weren't pinned down in some foxhole, and not one of us was going to die because of my poor judgment. Keep on keeping on!

I felt really bad about not being able to get my number-one buddy all the way to his home in northern Texas. I even tried to give him some of his money back but he wasn't about to take it. He just smiled and told me to hang onto it. He reminded me that I was not dead yet. Texas was coming up, and the way my car was acting I was bound to run out of money before the Great State of

Texas ran out of oil. The case of oil that had been in my trunk since we left California was dwindling, but there was enough to last us for a couple of hundred miles yet. I would get more soon.

Another young marine had made it home safe and sound by the time we reached Las Cruces, New Mexico, and he really was an extraordinarily happy camper. He was smiling from ear to ear as he pulled his sea bag out of the trunk of my car and said adios. The death of my car radio had been a big and unexpected disappointment, for sure. But I was ready for the oil problem and I still believed I could make it if I could only keep up with that situation. Like I said, empty oil can after empty oil can—no fun!

I was beginning to feel like a man shoveling sand against an incoming tide. Texas was getting closer by the mile, my case of motor oil had dwindled, and my passengers had dwindled also. Now there were only two ex-marines and one sailor. Texas had more oil than I could ever buy, that was true enough, and now it was looking as though all of the oil in Texas could not save my dreams. But like the man said, I was not dead yet!

After the sudden rainstorm we had left the top up. Our sailor boy had taken a piece of coat hanger out of his sea bag and he fashioned a hook of sorts out of it. The USMC calls that sort of thing "field expedience." The sailor called it damned good thinking. The device enabled him to hang his radio on the convertible top. We could hear the music a lot better, but soon the battery died and silence filled the empty space once more.

We made it to Roswell, New Mexico just in time to get another case of oil. I was laughing as I told my two remaining passengers that not one drop of oil would be bought by me in the Lone Star State. They could keep their damned oil. From Roswell, New Mexico to Lamesa, Texas, "I don't give a damn" was at the wheel, big time. That extra-clean Olds had gone through a case of motor oil traveling from California to New Mexico. Now it would use another half a case in less than half that distance. The death of my canary-yellow Oldsmobile looked to be a foregone conclusion at that point.

Driving like the madman that I was (Damn the torpedoes, full speed ahead!), every fifty miles I had to stop and pour another quart of oil into the black hole located on one of the valve covers. I was really getting tired of looking at that black, oil-drinking hole—man, was I ever! It was all I could do to keep my eyes open when I was behind the steering wheel. When I was not behind the wheel, which was far too often now, the fumes from the hot engine were so strong that they seemed to be both putting me to sleep and keeping me awake. I was even beginning to see some white smoke coming out of that black hole and drifting aimlessly past my squinted eyes. I knew exactly what that meant but I was determined not to dwell on that just yet!

Finally we drove into Lamesa just a bit shy of 3 A.M. on the morning of our fourth day. My number one buddy was closer to home than he had been in some time. I really did feel bad about the whole rotten trip. I'm sure he thought he knew just how bad I felt. One thing he didn't know was how much uncertainty and desperation was building up inside of me over the situation I would be faced with at the end of my journey.

I tried again to give him some money and once again he refused to take it. He told me that he hoped our paths crossed again one day and I was quick to agree. We shook hands and then the sailor who was standing outside the car with us beneath a big Lamesa, Texas street-light (everything is bigger in Texas, you know) shook his hand also. My number one buddy turned and walked off in the direction of an extra-large (once more) amber blinking traffic light. He didn't say it, but I knew he wanted to believe that my dream car was going to make it all the way to Miami, Florida. But that night, Kerrick, Texas was his destination and odds are that he made it home.

Prior to the injury to my brain a year later, I often thought about that guy. I wondered if he had ever been recalled by the corps and sent to 'Nam. The odds being what they were over there in that jungle, I can only hope that if he was recalled he made it home from that fight as well. Unfortunately, his name is one of those memories that seems to have been left on the side of the road with the oil cans. TBI does that.

I motioned for the sailor to take the wheel as I slid into the back seat. I was totally exhausted. I heard the US Navy slam both my trunk and my hood closed in that order. That was followed by the clunking sound of some empty oil cans as they skipped off into the thick Texas brush on the side of the road.

My dependable transportation was extremely undependable from the outset and I knew it. One big screw up! A fine way to get oneself headed in the direction of successful independence. The situation yet to be faced in North Miami Beach was intimidating in so many ways. Chicago would have been a lot better. But my dream car would have suffered the same death on Route 66, I'm sure. Maybe if I had gone to the Windy City at that time instead of going when I finally did, though, who knows? I might have missed TBI altogether.

That didn't happen! I had gambled with my newfound freedom and I had lost, big time. Just how big my loss would prove to be later on was the last question I had for myself before sleep swept me off to the land of whip and diddley. Swept me off, shoot! I was out before our last oil can bounced off the road.

We were now only about halfway across Texas. If a more southerly route like the one the map maker had devised in the first place had been taken and if, and if, and if...I could have been in Southern Alabama before the end of my fourth day of travel. Could'a, would'a, should'a.

Approximately 6 a.m. civilian time on the morning of the fifth day of my coast-to-coast excursion, I woke up to a smell I had become somewhat accustomed to after having spent three years of my life as a USMC mechanic: the good old smell of an internal combustion engine overheating. Yawning and stretching and setting forth a string of expletives that my mother's bar of soap would have turned red over, I was pleased to see that the navy still had someone doing the driving.

Glancing out of the window led me to the realization that we were in the Texas town called Sonora. Anything in any way resembling a gas station was what we needed to find, and fast! Our radiator was finally overheating big time. I detected a faint knocking sound as well.

It wasn't exactly a gas station we found, but it did have something resembling a gasoline pump standing out front. A big old dilapidated "machine shop" sign and some outdated farm equipment which was scattered around the apparent parking lot caused me to believe that some kind of help was on the premises. It looked as though some folks were just opening the place up for business.

We spotted a water spigot and an old rusty two-gallon tin can on the north side of the building. We both got out of the car quickly and I picked up a greasy-looking old rag off the ground. I successfully loosened the radiator cap with it. Hot water and steam spewed out in all directions, just missing both of us. My sailor-boy buddy had that rusty old can full of water and he was emptying it into the overheated radiator as I walked into the cinder block building. Yes sir. Field expedience or just damned good thinking, that sailor was on the ball. The loud knocking sound that the Olds engine had begun to make just as we pulled up to the water spigot seemed to be getting much louder.

Once inside the building, I was greeted by your everyday machinist-type individual, clad in a clean-looking pair of gray coveralls. Shortly before 7 a.m. on that Sonora, Texas morning, from beneath a red oil rag tucked into the back pocket of a gray pair of coveralls, came the wallet that would produce $100. That was all it took to make that lucky machinist the owner of my very clean, extra-shiny 1958 canary-yellow Oldsmobile convertible.

That whole episode reminds me of another quote from Shakespeare: "The coward dies a thousand deaths, the valiant, only once!" I indicated earlier that no one died trying to keep my dream car alive, but we all fought the good fight—even the sailor boy!

Believe me, in many ways I was pleased to be out from under that well-oiled machine. Pleased, perhaps, but undone nonetheless. Within a couple of hours, one worn-out sailor and one very disappointed ex- marine caught a ride to New Orleans, Louisiana. The sailor and I split up before we reached his destination. I was headed for the downtown Greyhound bus station, and he was headed for a different part of the city that he called his home. He went one way and I went the other. He was a good man—one of the navy's proudest!

As most any gambler will tell you, you never count your money when you're sitting at the table, and my money had not been counted since I left San Diego, California. But now that my gamble was done, I felt this strange urge to know exactly how much money I had left to my name. I had $322 in my wallet, and a little over $100 in my pocket, bringing my total worth to $422 and some change. In the bar room of the Greyhound bus station, $22 and change was more than enough to keep me entertained during my two-hour wait for a bus going to Florida.

When I woke up the next day on that southbound Greyhound, I was feeling a bit like a dog that had been run over by a bus myself. It was both unpleasant and embarrassing. The seat just behind the bus driver was occupied by yours truly and a large white pillow. I asked the driver where the pillow came from. He grinned, smiled, and laughed out loud. Then he told me that the folks that had put me on the bus had paid for it. It was no big surprise to me that I wasn't able to remember much about my time spent at the bar in the bus station, let alone boarding the bus. The pounding in my head had been telling me that I had really tied one on in that place.

Along with some people of color, three of whom were ex-marines also, I apparently had tried to drink all of the beer they had in the place. It was simply amazing, I thought. There I was, sitting at a bar in New Orleans and drinking beer with people who were my equals—no question about that. Yet these black people would not even have been allowed in the place six months prior to that day. It was a great time for us all to celebrate and it was absolutely a fine opportunity for us to solve the racial problems of the entire world.

Unknown to most folks, and right there in the Greyhound bus station in New Orleans, Louisiana in July of 1962, mankind truly became one people. Seven men—one white guy and six black guys, laughed, cried, raised glasses…and they all got me on the bus safely, soundly and on time. Martin Luther King would have been one extremely proud and happy camper that night in 1962. I was!

One week after leaving the marines I was looking for work and living with my mother and stepfather back in North Miami Beach. I had planned to stay with them for only a short time, hopefully just long enough to get my feet on the ground. Remember, I had some uncomfortable feelings about that situation.

I was paying my own way with what was left of the severance pay that I had received from the marines. It wasn't all that much by the time I finally got there, but at least I wasn't totally broke. I was able to find a few odd jobs as well, and that helped. All too soon, however, it became clear to me that my mother and stepfather were not that happy to have me around. The fact that the marines had made a man out of me was a big plus in that relationship, but you might say that it was apparent that too much water had gone over the dam earlier, during my high school days.

Transportation was the big issue. I just could not find a job without being able to get around the greater Miami area. In very short order it all came roaring back to me. I remembered why I had gone to "Paris" at the age of seventeen in the first place. No help, no support, nothing. Nothing! People who need people are what? Living with my mother and stepfather sure wasn't working out.

Finally I wrote a letter to the Engstroms at the suggestion of my mother, and sent it off post-haste. I had not thought about them in many, many moons. I guess I always had this crazy idea that home was where my mother was.

I asked the Engstroms for their help with my employment situation. They sent back a confirming letter and I was off. If only I could have caught a glimpse of the future, you can bet your boots I would have stayed put in North Miami Beach on that day regardless of any negative feelings I may have had at the time.

It seems to me that most of my decisions, especially early on in life, were made according to emotion rather than rational thinking. Not good! It's far too easy to blame everything that happens in life on someone else, isn't it? Shoot! I could blame just about every rotten thing that has happened in my life on someone else. Line them all up right now. But no can do. Most of them aren't even around to argue with me anymore in the first place. I win—by default!

The USMC teaches every marine how to deal with adversity: You simply fight it until you are victorious over it—victorious or dead, one or the other. You are a take-charge marine. You will kick ass and you WILL take names!

Yes, there are many ways to deal with adversity in life. My mother had her way, my father had his way, and the USMC definitely has their way. However, I have become convinced that there is only one way to completely overcome all of the adversity in life, and that is simply through faith and education. It certainly works for me now, today and every day.

With my USMC discharge and my 3516 (Automotive Mechanic Training Certificate) in hand, I was headed for the Windy City once more. I had not been in the Chicago area since 1952 when, for a brief time, my mother, my sister, and I had stayed in the home of an aunt and uncle in Fairview, Illinois after leaving Our Good Old LBO. While staying with them, and due to some very enterprising older cousins, I had become a caddy at the Butterfield Country Club—a small caddy but a caddy nonetheless. Anything that had to do with a ball, hitting or catching, was of great interest to me. Carrying a golf bag around for hours was only of minimal interest but the money was nice. Besides, many of the hackers (would-be golfers) asked especially for me, "the little blond kid that likes to shag golf balls by catching them in the air and then marking the spot with his skinny little frame." I loved to do that. Those guys always tipped well and they never asked me to carry their clubs either. A person can really learn to judge a fly ball by doing that for a few hours a day for a couple of months in succession.

Upon my return, Mrs. Engstrom, "Ma," seemed to pick up right where we left off so many years before. I remember her telling me once, back when I was still riding my tricycle up and down Mohawk Drive in Blackhawk Heights, that she was always going to have an extra-large place in her heart for her little Joey. (I hated that name!)

Unfortunately, my dog Pudge, rock hound extraordinaire, had passed away. Their beautiful daughter Mary Jo had married and had started a family of her own.

The Engstroms, both Ma and Pa, expressed a desire to help me get some sort of a life and future in place. They even had what they called their "extra" car, a good-looking and good-running, low-mileage 1957 Chevrolet that they insisted on giving to me. I in turn insisted that I would pay them for the car and my room and board just as soon as I possibly could.

Pa was in an administrative position at one of International Harvester's plants outside of Chicago. He had been with them for years. In no time at all he was able to line me up with a really good job—one with a future, paid vacations and all.

One evening, while sitting on the back porch that Pa had built for Ma as an anniversary present in 1948, we all had a really long, homespun conversation. Ma brought up the nicknames she used to call me ("Speed" and "Calamity Joe"), and I told them that both names had stuck to me like glue. From there, I went on to tell them about my speed, both in running and in throwing a ball, and how I had messed up my knee. I saw that as the biggest calamity of my life at that point, bar none! They actually listened to every word I said. The more interest they showed, the more I shared with them, including my dreams about baseball.

The very next day, a Saturday, Pa wanted to see me throw. He went to the trunk of his car and came back with two fairly old-looking softball gloves. He said he thought there was a baseball

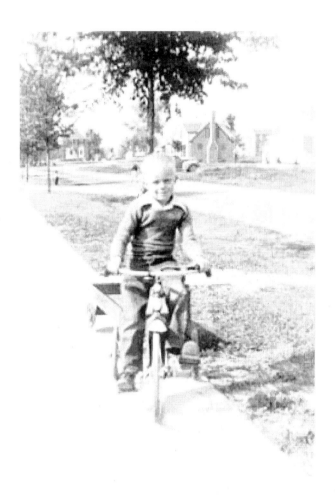

"Joey" Blakemore riding his tricycle. 1946.

in the basement that had been there for years as well. There was,

and Pudge must have retrieved it a couple of times at least. I could see the indentations her teeth had made in the hide.

We went out to the front yard. Pa awkwardly stepped off sixty feet, six inches, and handed me the ball. "Take it easy on me, Joe. I jus' wanna see a little bit."

"Don't worry," I said. "Just watch my form." I had absolutely no intention of throwing hard. The ball was really easy to grip thanks to good old Pudge. I went into my wind-up and made my usual long stride toward "the plate" (where Pa was standing, in this case). I felt the off-speed drop leave my fingertips. It wasn't all that super, but I knew right away by the look on his face that Pa was impressed.

"That was pretty darn good. Do they all do that?" He asked.

"Sure!" I replied. "If I throw 'em faster, I can make 'em do more 'n that."

That small amount of interest sure made me feel good—did it ever! For what was to be a very short time, I knew beyond a doubt that I had finally found the support I had been looking for. Boy, did I feel good, or what?! I even began to entertain some thoughts, here and there, and with considerable confidence I might add, about my covert operation. And now, with the belief I just knew these people had in me, I was homeward bound. (Get it? HOMEward bound.) Do you understand what I'm saying?

So, there I was back in Blackhawk Heights, with everything running along smoothly once again. My future looked absolutely bright. I loved living with these people. Hearing stories about my early childhood was great. Everything was really looking super. International Harvester was right up my alley and right in line with my USMC experience. I was becoming extremely happy because everything seemed to be going my way. I almost felt as though I had never left the Engstroms' home at all. My knee was getting a lot better, or so I wanted to think, anyway.

I was sure my fast ball had gotten even faster since I'd left Okinawa, and it had been a blazer before. (In the corps I had been throwing consistently on the high side of eighty miles per hour.) I guess the few pounds I had managed to put on since leaving the Rock had given me a little extra pop. I wanted to believe that my drop was really dropping as straight down as it ever had and that it was moving around really well. (The baseball people of today don't call what I was throwing back then a drop. I believe today they call it a slider. As my son likes to say, "Whatever!") As many baseball people say, I was coming straight over the top with excellent control.

My confidence was high even if my knee was less than 100 percent. I figured I was not going to be doing too many things that would cause my knee to go out. All I really wanted to do was show off my throwing ability. I could still bring the ball (throw it hard), super feeling or no super feeling. Of course, that supernatural feeling was long gone. I had convinced myself that a tryout would go just great with or without it. And I knew the Engstroms were on my side. They even suggested I let their doctor take a look at my troubled left knee.

Playing baseball, preferably for the Chicago Cubs...what a dream! Dream, shoot! It was my supernatural reality. You can bet your last pair of spikes on that. I was not about to throw in the towel when it came to the game of baseball. It was my destiny, after all. Wrigley Field, here I come.

I had gotten Hank Sauer's and Clyde McCullough's autographs there years before. Hank was a left fielder and Clyde was a catcher. Both of them were playing in the first big league baseball game I had ever seen. All of the boys in the LBO (no girls allowed—that's how things worked in the olden days, you know!) got to go to downtown Chicago to see the Cubs hopefully whip up on the Milwaukee Braves. (No, I did not misspeak. Back then they really were the Milwaukee Braves, not the Brewers.)

The Cubs lost that day, and the next day, and the next as well. The Cubs have been getting whipped for years. (But listen up! We're still cheering them Cubbies on down here, Harry. I promise!)

As I thought about my intentions of trying out for the Chicago Cubs, I also thought about what Mantle and Berra had done with the New York Yankees some years earlier. I had heard (I didn't know for sure), that Mickey and Yogi had simply asked for tryouts and they got them. The rest was history. Of course, Yogi Berra and Mickey Mantle were not pitchers, and both had good knees at the time.

Sure, I knew then and I know now that every other male child dreams of becoming a major league ballplayer at some time in his life. To be a great athlete of some kind—any kind! For me, playing baseball just came naturally, and many people had seen my talent. The time finally looked right to move baseball to a front burner.

CHAPTER 6

Paradoxical Ambiguity

When I stop to think about the war in Vietnam, I realize the magnitude of it all when measured in lost lives. A sea of bald-headed United States Marines marches across my mind. Baseball and my knee injury seem trivial at best.

You might say, and rightly so more than likely, that I'm lucky to be alive because of both baseball and my weak left knee. You might say Lady Luck was looking out for me, for sure. I had served my country honorably. I had a good job, a fine place to live, and what appeared to be a great-looking future, even if I never did get to play professional baseball. The Engstroms' home and International Harvester were a long way from 'Nam and harm's way.

If indeed it was just plain old luck that kept me from being wasted in some rice paddy in 'Nam, then luck certainly deserted me on that hot August night in 1963 on Butterfield Country Club Road.

Once upon a time, back in the early '50s, back before there were golf carts, I had worked as a very young caddy at the Butterfield Country Club. But on this warm night, the third day of August, 1963, almost 14 years after my Lake Bluff experience, and almost one year to the day from my separation from active duty in the USMC, near that same large golf course, I was a passenger in a 1959 Hot Rod Chevy.

Like all too many young people back then (and now as well), the youthful driver of that extra-clean-looking Hot Rod knew only two speeds: very fast and sudden stop. I loved the fast part. But stop we did, with the front bumper and left front fender mashed and folded up against one very large elm tree.

I was unconscious and semi-conscious for twenty-eight days, and have had one gigantic hangover for the past forty years—no lie! I had had way too much to drink at a party before I ever climbed into that Hot Rod Chevy. You might say I threw my life away for a dozen cans of beer. How smart was that? Not very, was it?

I regained consciousness only to be told that I would never again be the same as I had been before that warm and dreadful August night. I would not realize the awful truth of that statement for many years to come. As a matter of fact, I'm still realizing what that means with every key I push on this keyboard.

The prognosis was simple: brain damage. The effects were not so simple. Not by a long shot. I was not expected to ever walk, talk, see, or be in any way the person I had come to be over the preceding twenty-two years of my life.

The changes I was going to go through for the rest of my life were simply beyond my comprehension. Basically, I was one big neurological mess, indeed. As I said, I was told that I would never walk, talk, or see correctly again. I do and I don't. I will and I won't. I have and I have not.

Only another survivor of TBI can come close to a genuine understanding of the preceding paragraph. Empathy, the true participation in another's feelings or ideas, is difficult at best, but empathy is a word that many head injury survivors simply don't care to hear anymore.

What I suffered as a result of my auto accident was being referred to at that time as irreversible and residual brain damage. The impact of my head striking the rearview mirror of the car I was riding in was so great that it displaced all of the fluid that my brain, just like yours, floats in. This displacement of fluid allowed my brain to smash into the inside of my skull with enough force to both bruise and destroy precious brain cells. If you're interested in more general information about TBI in the present day, you may want to look at appendices A, B, and C. But the important thing worth remembering about my experience in 1963 is that back then seat belts were not at all cool. So much for being cool.

When I did finally regain full consciousness, I found myself in a large room. Flowers were everywhere. It took me days if not months to figure out exactly who and where I was. I thought I could understand what people around me were saying, but for some strange reason I was not communicating with them well at all. The woman standing beside my bed looked somewhat familiar to me, but I was simply not sure who she was. Everything I tried to look at seemed somehow familiar yet very different.

When the person standing next to my bed began speaking, she told me who she was. Pauline Engstrom was her name, and my name was Joe Blakemore. Any recollection of having ever called this person "Ma" was simply gone, but looking back it seems fitting somehow that she, the woman who had provided me with a real sense of family, would be the one who was there by my side.

I was in the Elmhurst General Hospital in Elmhurst, Illinois, just a few miles outside of the Big Windy, Shy Town, Chicago. Ever so slowly, I began to understand about the flowers in the room. Strange as it may seem to someone who has never had his or her bell rung really well, I was having a real problem with all of those darn flowers. On top of that, it took every bit of two weeks at least before I even realized I had double vision. Everything around me was double. At least that's how I saw everything. It took me quite a while to figure out that by closing one eye I could see things a bit better. Even then I had to be reminded of that fact many times by others. I also had some paralysis of the left side of my face and left extremities, mild amnesia, aphasia and, oh yes, something called diplopia, which was what was playing tricks with my vision.

Diplopia, in lay terminology, is seeing double. I have since had an operation on my eyes for the correction of diplopia (it's interesting when I realize that my first operation of this type took place fifteen years after the onset of my injuries in 1963), and to some degree the operation was successful. At this time I only see double at certain angles, although this can be problematic. But like TBI in general, you can learn to live with it. You should never forget that God created humans to be the most adaptable of all organisms.

Again in layman's terms, and I'm quoting a doctor here, "Aphasia is like when you ask someone to hand you a broom and they hand you a mop. In reality you have been handed a mop because that is exactly what you have asked for." Believe me, many times over the years I have been positive that I have said one thing only to be told that I had said something totally different. Think about it for a minute. In the lives of most "normal" normal people (I use the term normal awfully loosely here), when something like that occurs, it almost always results in some type of conflict. Conflict after conflict has resulted from my aphasia, and in any real context I have always been the one who was wrong. Learning to live with aphasia has been extraordinarily challenging. Learning to use aphasia in any way that will lead to a positive and favorable outcome is absolutely divine.

It's difficult for me, in some cases impossible, to recall much of what took place during my six-month stay in Elmhurst General. I was totally unaware of who was or was not there, or so most people thought at that time.

As for knowing who I was and where I was and what the flowers were all about (even though this seemingly very nice person had told me over and over again), well, that became clearer and clearer to me as the days and weeks passed.

And you're probably wondering exactly what happened to the driver of that Hot Rod Chevy. I don't know now, and I REALLY didn't know then. And in addition, thinking about that now is something I'd rather not do.

With the passage of time and the help of others, I have been able to reconstruct some of what took place in that hospital. Today, at the age of sixty-two, recalling and reconstructing my stay seems to be easier and more accurate than ever before. All sorts of things continue to come to my mind—things that I had zero recollection of until recently. Strange stuff like that can keep me entertained endlessly—it's better than TV!

For some reason I think I can remember walking out of the ambulance and into a small room in the hospital. At that moment it seems to me that I was walking and talking just fine. I absolutely believe I was standing there talking to some emergency room attendants when, just like that, my lights went out and they have never come back on completely to this day. One huge hangover, for sure!

I think I remember falling in love with a nurse. It seems to me this particular nurse would often hold my hand and talk to me until I was overcome by sleep. She expressed the desire to take care of me for the rest of my life. Whatever happened with that situation is beyond my memory.

I'm sure I remember the day President Kennedy was shot. Strange, but true. Or maybe it's like something that's been told to you over and over again until you think you remember it. I'm not sure. One thing I am sure of: We all may have been better off in many ways if someone had simply canceled 1963.

My speaking ability was practically nonexistent. The first time I attempted to order someone around in my best, most positive and commanding tone, USMC all the way, while I was still flat on my back in a hospital bed was a real revelation. Believe me, I understood the concept of giving orders only too well, but this sounded to me like a voice that I had become familiar with at the age of four. I was so surprised at how silly I sounded that I burst into laughter. The laughter sounded odd and strangely silly to me as well.

The nurse who had been the intended target of my commands seemed unfazed by these orders and what had appeared to me to be some very weird-sounding laughter. I attempted to apologize for my outburst but she insisted that she hadn't any idea what I was talking about.

Knowing or understanding exactly what I was or was not aware of was difficult at best and most of the time it was impossible. Imagine being told that you don't know what you are doing or saying because you have injured your brain. Then imagine the same people telling you that there isn't any way for you or anyone else to know to what extent this is true or how long it will last or how often it will occur. Constantly being told you have forgotten something or that you said or did something that you have absolutely no recollection of can quickly become one big can of worms.

My behavior seemed to be questioned at all times, and at all times I absolutely believed I was doing just fine. Please don't get the wrong idea. I was told and I did accept the fact that I had severely injured my brain. I knew I was "not right." How "wrong" was I? How often was I wrong? How long would I be wrong?

The abstract thinking processes that I have had to acquaint or reacquaint myself with since my accident have led me to believe that there exists a shark-like mentality in many people. That old "kick them when they're down" feeding frenzy. If what I'm about to say sounds the least bit cynical to you, please accept my apologies, but I often wonder how many times I have been falsely accused. I'm not going to name names here, but I could.

Questioning my awareness has become second nature. I almost want to tell you that it's made me a much nicer guy. There is just no telling what it could do for the "normal" normal person. My abstract thinking ability has at least tripled since my injury, and that can be documented. Do I need documentation?

The path of least resistance was one that I definitely was not given the luxury of traveling. If I ever expected to loose the bonds of TBI, I was going to have to learn to accept the hard way, the way of being misunderstood, or "paradoxical ambiguity," as I sometimes like to refer to it. ("It" being the overall effects of TBI, of course.)

Did I have enough self-awareness and self-direction to choose the right course for my recovery? Could I choose a course that would lead to adjustment, adaptability and some type of self-acceptable recovery, at least? I thought I could, but most everyone else I knew seemed to have their doubts. Remember, there were few answers to those questions at that time. Many of those questions had yet to be formulated. The average person in 1963 didn't know what to ask, let alone how to respond to those important questions.

I was a very headstrong young man who had suddenly become lacking in many areas. Determination was definitely not one of those areas, so into the fray I went. I fought and I fought against the resistance. It was as though I had to learn how to do everything, even the simplest things, all over again. Buttons were one big pain in the butt. Shoelaces were out of the question. I'm sure that if loafers had not already been in existence I would have invented them. Velcro had not yet made its debut. My mind was willing to do most anything I had to do, but I seemed to be in some strange disconnect mode most of the time. I can only describe myself as being disconnected within and without. I was dizzy periodically, and off balance constantly, dizzy or not. I had slurred speech as well.

One day my doctor and a couple of his nurses brought me a mirror and a tube of lipstick. They were trying to ascertain just how much control I had over my upper extremities, but the simple task of putting lipstick on was impossible for me to accomplish. I had zero experience in the application of lipstick anyway. Not many men in that day and age did. One would have thought, however, that even a person without any prior knowledge of lipstick whatsoever would have at least been able to hold the mirror still and press the tube to his lips. Wave the mirror around? I did. Press the lipstick to every part of my face including my lips? I did. Hand/eye coordination? Poor at best. Lipstick waving as freely as that mirror? You bet. Appearing like a wild Indian who has gotten extremely carried away with the war paint ritual? You know it.

I broke into my nonsensical and uncontrollable laugh. The nurses in the room didn't seem to know whether to laugh or cry at first. One of them latched onto my mirror just before it flew out of my freely waving hand. I guarantee you that before they finished their little experiment I had all of them laughing, including the doctor who just happened to get hit in the chest with a lipstick tube.

But the whole thing was far from being funny. It was downright humiliating for me. I'm not really sure why all I could do at that time was laugh about it. It would take me another fifteen years to learn anything at all about the benefit of laughing at myself.

Satire is one of the things every TBI survivor should be told about as soon as is feasible after they experience their injury. I believe that the ability to laugh at oneself is priceless. Many "normal" normal people don't know when it is appropriate to laugh at themselves and when it is not. That's a shame! For TBI survivors, it's appropriate at all times. Who said "laugh and the world laughs with you, cry and you cry alone"? Had I known at the time what a good laugh at oneself does for a person, I'm confident that I would not have spent so many years crying and feeling sorry for myself. What a waste of time that was. Remember, I'm forty years post and I'm still laughing somehow. Laughing really seems important to me. Of course, taking the feelings of other people into consideration even when you have every reason not to is equally important.

Along with the understanding of who and where I was came the understanding that I was a former United States Marine. A former Marine who finds himself in such a predicament says to himself, in no uncertain terms, "How in the hell do I get out of this place?"

I believe it is very important to understand that the question was "How do I get out?" and not "How did I get in?" The point is that at all times one should separate the negative from the positive, and, as Johnny Mercer said, "Don't mess with Mister In-between."

To any good "Jar Head" (and my head was definitely ajar, pardon the pun), escape was the only positive venture. There isn't any in-between to consider. I could not tell you much, if anything, about my experience with the marines at that time. I didn't even know I had been one until I was told. However, what the corps had instilled in that seventeen-year-old kid some years prior was some extremely tough and powerful stuff. That good old can do attitude has been there for me on more than one occasion in my life.

Yes, I did try to escape from the hospital one time and only one time. Once was more than enough. My bed was right next to a window facing the street. If I closed one eye, my double vision was gone. The elimination of my double vision by no means took care of my sight problems altogether. Every once in a while, though, I could see what appeared to be a city bus going by. I was sure I was seeing that bus better and better all the time.

After a couple of months, my left leg began to feel a bit more like it was there again. I guess I was just not convinced about what everyone was telling me regarding my ability, or my lack of ability, to walk. So, in spite of my vertigo, dizziness, overall feeling of weakness, and this horrendous feeling of disconnectedness, and without making any plans, I simply felt myself sliding over the side of the bed feet first, dangling, and reaching for that big, very clean-looking, bright concrete floor.

My first step living with TBI was a big discouragement at best. Nothing. Nothing was there, no real feeling—a very strange sensation, for sure. Fortunately, albeit unpleasantly, I landed on my butt, not on my head. The sound of stainless steel pans hitting the floor along with me was not at all pleasant, either. Everyone had been telling me the truth. And to add to my embarrassment, one partially full urinal and one bedpan, also in need of emptying, came crashing down alongside me. There I was, lying flat on my back on that (not so clean anymore) big gray floor.

The nurses (good-looking nurses!) could not have missed hearing the commotion. I had never received that much attention in my entire life. They had me back in bed in record time, and before you could say Jackie Robinson (or, for the younger generation, Dion Sanders), the big gray floor was clean once more. The only real damage that had been done was to my pride.

That wonderful person in my life, Ma, Pauline Engstrom, was there in plain view, standing next to my bed, reminding me once more that I was absolutely not in heaven, especially not at that moment. She was right. At that particular moment, I was absolutely NOT in heaven. I'm convinced that at that moment I had been much closer to a permanent hell than at any other time in my life. I felt as though I was on the outskirts of hell. TBI, traumatic brain injury, the state of TBI, was definitely a type of hell from which there was no escape. Absolutely no escape. But with God, all things are possible.

So ended my one and only attempt to escape from the hospital.

That was not the first time that the lady standing at my bedside had to make it clear to me that I had not died and gone to heaven. I had first suspected that that was where I was because of all of the flowers surrounding my bed and all of my other strange and altered perceptions, not to mention that huge white throne I had been standing before for what seemed to me to be forever.

No one else saw that big throne or me standing before it. Be that as it may, I believe to this day, simply no question about it, that I was standing before a huge and very bright white throne and that I was given a second chance at life. If I could explain what I have just claimed in a more acceptable way, believe me, I definitely would, but I can't. And I can't say that I've done a lot better with the second chance than I did with the first. It has become crystal clear to me since then, however, that my acceptance of Christ as my Lord and Savior was something that I had to do in order to escape both a living hell and an eternal hell as well, but it would take another ten years of needless suffering before I did just that.

I have always believed that without my God-given athletic ability and Christ in my life, I would have never moved in the right direction—I could never have come this far in my attempts to overcome TBI, and everything I have experienced in my far-out life would have been much harder to deal with.

On the other hand, being an athlete and then suddenly being faced with a lifetime of physical limitations can be a huge psychological blow. I had really developed an attitude about my ability to play the game of baseball at a young age. God had given it to me. There wasn't a man alive who could take it from me. I had kept somewhat of a low profile regarding my abilities until I was in my early twenties, not because I wanted to, necessarily, but because the opportunity and the timing never seemed right. Physical maturity did seem to be occurring a little slower for me than it did for the average boy my age. I was very much aware of my youthful appearance and had accepted it as a good thing. There was not a single doubt in my mind. I was going to play baseball, big time, sooner or later.

How about never?! Would never be too soon? What a shocking revelation. Brain damage. TBI. Ouch. I would never be able to play ball again. All my athletic ability was gone for good. I was absolutely blown away. Why me, God? Why me? "Never put all of your eggs in one basket, kid," resounded over and over in my mind. The best-laid plans are made by whom? Who makes the best plans, Mr. Steinbeck?

Remembering the day a nurse took me to the large physical therapy room in the hospital, a room that appeared to me to be some sort of a padded or "rubber room", always reminds me how far I have come in my never-ending recovery. This was the first time that I had been out of my hospital bed in four months with the exception of my unsuccessful escape attempt. The large PT room was similar to a room used to detain a person who may have flown entirely too high over the cuckoo's nest. My therapy nurse, who just happened to bear a strange resemblance to one of my old USMC drill instructors from my yesteryears, ordered me to begin crawling around on the floor of this room, which was covered with large gray mats. The idea, she explained in her masculine, ice-cold and stoic tone of voice, was simply that if I ever wanted to learn to walk again, learning to crawl was essential. She really did come across like a Marine Corps drill instructor. I was being told in no uncertain terms that I had to learn to crawl allover again. I was not being given any choice in the matter whatsoever. I would learn to crawl or else. Inquiring about the "or else" part of it did not interest me at all—not one bit. I really didn't care to hear it. I certainly did not want any part of it, but like it or not, this type of hell was my new reality. For some seemingly unexplainable reason, though, I have always had the idea that this type of hell was far better than the one I had almost wound up in.

Crawling was far from easy for me to accomplish and simply trying to crawl was absolute hell for sure. Teaching me to crawl was my new DI's top priority, and learning how to crawl soon became mine as well. Simply being in the presence of my physical therapy nurse was hell as well. Life for me was beginning to look like one big obstacle course indeed. I remember how surprising it was for me to realize that I was unable to crawl in the first place.

Not being able to crawl due to my head injury was far from my only problem. I soon realized that anything I did, including sitting motionless in my wheelchair, was accompanied by a terrible feeling. That terrible feeling defies all human explanation. In my case there has always been a persistent feeling of disconnectedness and confusion. Although this has noticeably diminished over time, it has remained unexplainable to a great degree.

Any attempt to explain my feeling of disconnectedness to anyone else over the years has always wound up being ambiguous and paradoxical. Yet my explanation has, beyond a doubt, been my reality.

My balance was so badly impaired that I could not maintain it even on my hands and knees. It took a lot of repetition, but my combat-boots-type nurse ultimately taught me to crawl once more without any help from anyone. Accomplishing the crawling challenge did give me a glimmer of hope.

I think I also remember an older guy, an apparent stroke victim, who was about the same age as I am today. After my routine crawling attempts one afternoon, some therapy attendants had put me back into a wheelchair. I overheard this older fellow slurring every word he spoke. His ability to speak was poor, but in many was mine was even worse. Listening to him trying to say anything was really hard for me. I attempted to ignore the man altogether.

Being ignored is another one of the things a TBI victim must learn to deal with. Dealing with being ignored has definitely made me a much better person, but there is a lot to be said for the shoe being on the other foot. Anyway, what that older guy was trying hard to tell the nurse as she helped him hold onto the rail while he walked around the PT room was that I was a really lucky kid.

(That rail, by the way, due to my double vision, neurological confusion and what I call disconnectedness, seemed to have neither a beginning nor an end. My visual perception was extremely unusual, to say the least. Gray mats appeared to be everywhere—literally everywhere!)

I overheard that older guy trying to tell his nurse that in twenty years or so I wouldn't even know such a thing had ever happened to me. Of course, the older fellow didn't really know what he was talking about, and ignoring him as it turns out was the best thing for me to do. I didn't realize that at the time, however. I just couldn't stand hearing him try to talk about anything at all, right or wrong! He was much too hard to listen to, and besides, twenty years in my condition or anything close to it was out of the question, or so I wanted to think, anyway. Thanks but no thanks! Even if the guy had been speaking plainly I sure didn't care to listen to what he was saying.

At this time, forty years post TBI, I still believe luck has had absolutely noting to do with anything in my life. The man was wrong about that. But nevertheless I try awfully hard not to ignore anyone anymore. Even when folks try to tell me how lucky I am today, I listen but I know better! The number of times my speech has caused me not to be heard is countless. Each time I have become aware of not being listened to, and have accepted the fact, another lesson has been learned.

Listening is one of our most powerful human abilities. I can say that firsthand and without any reservation. I know that on many occasions I have literally forced myself to listen and to trust my damaged brain. The power I have personally derived from listening has been nothing short of fantastic.

TBI survivors who are capable of knowing what I'm talking about definitely have a leg up on their recovery. But if you can't listen, can't retain, can't remember, can't walk, talk, or see correctly, then try, try again!

I recall making up a little song to the dismay of many of the people around me. I would sing it on my worst days, when my mind or body showed extreme signs of being stubborn and non-responsive. "If you really don't want to do it, just go ahead and do it anyhow." I sang that little one-line masterpiece over and over again. It really did help me a lot at the time.

My new crawl was awkward, and it was never going to be the crawl it had been once upon a time, but it did become good enough in time to allow me to take a shot at the next big challenge: walking, of course.

The meaning of putting one foot in front of the other became crystal clear to me. I was experiencing concentration on a new level. It was as though I had to concentrate extra hard in order to do most anything I tried to do. Moving my feet was no exception! Many of the things that had become second nature to me by that time in my life were very difficult to do. I had to be reminded to concentrate over and over again. At the same time there was this crazy, and I do mean crazy, problem with my self-awareness. An on again, off again type of scenario. Crazy!

Before I left Elmhurst General I could stand and take a couple of steps with some assistance. Awkward and assisted, yes, but every step was a true milestone in my thinking. It seemed very odd to me the way other people seemed far less impressed with both my walking and my crawling.

I cannot tell you how to overcome brain damage any more than I can tell you how to survive a rattlesnake bite. But I can tell you how I did it, and I have done it! One thing I have learned along the way is that success is really hard to argue with.

On my hospital medical chart the words were there for anyone to see: "Not recommended for rehabilitation." If head injury survivors buy into not being able to do something, then they won't ever do it! That's applicable to most of the "normal" normal folks that I have met in my lifetime as well.

CHAPTER 7

Attacking in Another Direction

My sister Judy, to this very day, tells me that she couldn't understand why my mother and stepfather, at least my mother anyway, could not find the time to fly to Chicago right after they got word of the accident. Judy was awfully upset over the fact that she could not fly up, but at that time she was pregnant with her first child. Back then, few pregnant women were allowed to board an airplane. Apparently my sister's pregnancy was the justification my mother used for not being there herself.

I'm not at all sure that the presence of anyone in particular would have mattered to me all that much anyway. I really didn't know who or where I was at the time. Of course, doctors today tell us that that sort of thing matters a great deal to a TBI survivor.

I find it difficult to say that either one of my parents was absolutely wrong for not being by my bedside after my accident. I had been making my own choices in my life for quite a while. I had, perhaps, chosen to dance once too often. Sure enough, just as I had always been told, "If you dance, you've got to pay the piper." The day you become totally dependant on other people is the day you might fully understand the idea of paying the piper. The true importance of understanding other people's priorities might land squarely on your doorstep also.

After leaving the hospital in Elmhurst, Illinois, I was flown back, via Delta Airlines, to Miami International Airport. I would be staying once again with my mother and stepfather in North Miami Beach. Miami was definitely the last place on the face of planet earth that I wanted to go, but I was absolutely unable to stop it from happening. The Engstroms could not take care of me in their home. Their hands were tied by some unforeseen circumstances. It seems that while I was stuck in Elmhurst General Hospital, one of their elderly parents had become awfully sick and had to be moved into their home and cared for around the clock. I was a very sick person myself, both mentally and physically. I can only thank God that I never had bladder or bowel dysfunctions after leaving the hospital, so I did not need someone to look after me "twenty-four/seven." I did, however, have to accept the fact that wherever I was sent was where I was going to be.

That extremely significant person in my life, Ma, Pauline Engstrom, would be looking after me on the flight from Chicago's O'Hare airport. I don't even remember boarding the plane. I was out like a light the entire flight.

Although I didn't find this out until many years later, my estranged father was working as a head chef there at O'Hare on the very day of my flight back to nothing, absolutely nothing. Nothing was there. No real emotion. A very strange sensation. I was helpless, and considered by many people to be hopeless as well. Helpless and hopeless—now that's a real winning combo. My mother and stepfather did not have a clue as to what they could do for me, or with me for that matter, when I wound up back in their home. They accepted as being true what they were told by friends, relatives, and a limited number of doctors: not much hope, period. It's hard for me to say this, but sometimes I really wonder about their true concern.

And I can't say that Sir Donald ever even knew anything about my head injury. He died of liver complications a few years later at the age of fifty-three. Bright and functional he was, but alcohol finally did him in well before his time. He was one of life's losers. Very sad. Very sad, indeed.

A large part of the ongoing recovery of any head injury survivor is learning to accept the wrong end of the stick and make it work. Something like making lemonade out of a lemon. Take, for instance, what I said earlier: Where I was sent is where I was going to be. The priorities of the people where I would be sent offered me very little inner peace, if any at all. I had never found peace in that household, even before my misfortune. My mother definitely always had her own priorities. Everyone had priorities, and it appeared to me that all of my priorities had been forfeited to a very large degree after my accident.

When a person awakens to a life of TBI, all things are changed. Most everything will be constantly changing in many ways from that day on. In my case, even after gaining a good deal of my awareness back, I would be living in an altered state of consciousness for years to come. The things I found myself accepting due to my dependence on others were tough, but learning to question my own awareness of practically everything was even tougher.

I had some big problems. Some of those problems I still have today. At first, if I walked at all I had to use a walker, and I hated that. The best thing for me to do was to ride in a wheelchair. I hated that as well. My speech was a mess. I was constantly being told by others that I had said one thing when I was sure I had said another. I was given to involuntary muscle spasms which were a lot like a mild epileptic seizure. They were subject to occur at any time.

I soon found out that damage to my big USMC pride would be an ongoing occurrence. When it comes to landing on one's butt, for example, I have definitely gained a great deal of insight over the years. On more than one occasion I have found myself, without any apparent reason, sitting squarely on my posterior. Picture yourself, if you will, standing and talking to a friend one minute, and then suddenly dropping to your butt in a sitting position the next. Add to that the lack of an explanation for what has just taken place, other than hearing yourself say, "brain damage." More than embarrassing. I'm still occasionally subject to impromptu sitting. In five years time I had learned to fall so gracefully that I could do it in slow motion. I'm not kidding. I absolutely refused to use my walker, and I did fall often in what appeared to be some type of suspended animation. I have witnesses. (Do I need witnesses?) Anyway, my mother was somewhat successful at keeping me on my feet most of the time when she was around. When she was not around (most of the time I was left to my own devices) I fell many times. But I have learned two positive things about falling, whether it is in slow motion or not. First: getting back on my feet has become easier with every fall I have experienced. Second: living with embarrassment won't kill you.

Like most TBI survivors, I have been somewhat accident-prone at times—more often than not! Like the day I overheated the Wesson oil in the fish cooker. I can't remember what I did wrong. The Wesson oil I was using to cook my fish on that fine spring day reached its flash point, and bingo! Third degree burns over one third of my body.

Both of my legs were badly burned, and demanded a twenty-eight-day stay in the hospital—twenty-eight days of extreme consciousness this time. Skin grafts, hydrotherapy…not a fun time. My wife told my doctor, a burn specialist extraordinaire, that she "hoped I had learned my Wesson." I had to sell my fish cooker right away, but you know she made me do it. I did, however, write down how to do it the right way after that experience, so, you know, I'm ready just in case my wife lets me play with fire again one day.

I do, at times, turn short when aiming for a door opening, and slam into the door jamb. Hard-to-deal-with situations in anyone's life can be the most productive situations of all, but it's hard to find anything productive about slamming oneself into a door jamb.

Neglect is the word used to describe my aforementioned neurological problem with door jambs. Heightened awareness and extreme concentration have proven to be the key to success here, but at first they were out of reach and impossible for me to accomplish. Some of us simply have to work a lot harder at being normal. If you have "drain bamage" (sorry, I mean brain damage) you might convince me that you actually know what I'm saying.

By refusing to accept this new set of facts that were confronting me, self-pity was unavoidable. Deep down inside, I was developing this unforgiving hate for myself and everything else. My emotions, if I had any, were strange and different. I thought I knew what I was supposed to be feeling in different situations and I would often find myself acting toward that end, but many times, in the middle of what I perceived to be an emotional situation, I would burst into uncontrollable laughter. There have also been many times, while engaged in conversation with someone, when I would feel my face contort as though I were about to cry. Over what, I haven't a clue. I have had to work on my strange lack of emotion and at the same time fight off over-exuberance and involuntary expression. There were many times when my emotions were obviously out of control and inappropriate.

There has been a degree of difficulty, beyond the norm, to everything I have done for the past forty years. I have experienced life in what I can only describe as a totally off-balanced state. Disconnected. At the time I also had this awful, uncomfortable and extremely strange feeling that's very difficult for me to explain. It was as though I was in a fish bowl looking out. I could see everyone and everyone could see me; however, successfully interacting with other people on any level, especially cultivating new friendships, was next to impossible. The cultivation of friendships remains difficult for me to this very day, even though I do spend far less time in that fish bowl.

I have always felt strangely lacking in my communication attempts, and no one ever seemed to be able to help me out of that fish bowl that I mentioned above. With the exception of a few neurological professionals, no one seemed to even have much interest in my fish bowl. If I tried to explain, I soon found that I might as well sign my own declaration of insanity.

Throughout my never-ending recovery, I have found myself asking the same question of anyone and everyone, much too often: "Do you understand what I'm saying?" I have even asked it of you, the reader, once or twice. Asking that question of many supposedly intelligent medical people (actually egotistical clowns for the most part) did not help my cause much at all along the way. I have yet to meet a person who was spouting off about being able to empathize with me, who ever really knew or cared much about what size moccasin I had worn into his or her office. Do you understand what I'm saying? I wish I had a dime for every time I've asked that question. In today's world, one should certainly wish for a dollar instead of a dime.

I have always been able to communicate and interact better with the people I had known before TBI. They always seemed to have a more in-depth and accurate understanding of all of the changes I was faced with. At the same time, having that understanding and having the desire or ability to cope with my new behavior proved to be impossible for almost everyone.

The rumor that I had a steel plate in my head seemed to spread like wildfire. Of course, I really didn't. I've never even had brain surgery. At the time, a closed head injury such as mine was better off remaining closed. In other words, my skull had not been fractured. I simply had brain damage. (Brain damage! Look out for that guy. We can't do anything with him—he's an extremely dangerous person.) And on top of that, I was an ex-marine at what seemed to be the wrong time in our country's history. You know, the 'Nam stigma. What a killer combination! But I'm not at all dangerous. I never really was a dangerous person in the first place. Yet I managed to alienate most of my old friends during the first eight years of my recovery.

A neurologist informed me one day that being steadfast and firm in to my opinions was a trait associated with TBI. Believe me, traits associated with TBI are a dime a dozen, and you certainly don't need any of them in your background. I always felt that his statement devalued my opinion and left me feeling uncomfortable and angry. If I really give it some thought, though, I'm sure that throughout my recovery attempt it has always been statements like his that have led me to value liberty the way I now do.

I really like what Mrs. Mill's son, John Stuart Mill, said in his book *On Liberty* in 1859: "If all mankind minus one were of one opinion, and only one person were of the contrary opinion, mankind would be no more justified in silencing that one person than he, if he had the power, would be justified in silencing mankind."

Yes, I am a very opinionated person. I'm proud of it, too. I believe that everyone should be very opinionated. Having your own opinion regarding anything and everything under the sun, and having the right to express that opinion, are truly precious liberties. I believe that as each one of us grows older we should attempt to express our opinions to everyone for their consideration. After all, you never know when your opinion might just prove to be extraordinary. To me, it seems a huge waste for us to go through life without forming opinions about the things we have learned. As for my opinions in general…well, I believe I have learned to suffer my opinions prior to giving them, solicited or unsolicited. As for the traits associated with TBI, I have found most of them to be extremely devaluating. However, with God's help I am successfully overcoming every one of them. Every single one.

The new friends I was making in North Miami Beach all seemed to bring with them a cure for all of our ills—theirs and mine. Flower power, pot, and lots of love. "All you need is love." It took me much too long to realize that love without God is simply no love at all.

My sexual needs were very hard to deal with. What compounded my situation was the simple fact that I had never been told what to expect pertaining to sexual behavior after TBI. Talking about sex in my home was strictly taboo back then. I was very confident about the fact that I was not at all homosexual, but at the same time I was confounded by some of my thinking. No one seemed to have any answers when it came to my situation at that time.

Most people who sustain TBI are left in either a hypersexual or a hyposexual state. Of course, I knew nothing of this at the time, and for many years I believed myself to be just another exceptionally normal ex-marine. As a matter of fact, I did not know anything contrary to that until a few years ago. My life would have been a lot less complicated if I had found out about "hyper" and "hypo" early on.

Dating was always a bad experience, at least for the first decade after the onset of my injury. The first time I went out with a member of the opposite sex was about three years after my accident. The sister of a good friend went with me to see a movie. She had told her brother that she liked me a lot. It took me a while, but finally I did ask her out. She drove. Once we arrived at the movie theater, I was so busy concentrating on my walking and my balance, while at the same time trying to hide my fish bowl, that I completely lost all awareness of much else. I was so happy to finally sit down in that theater seat, and of course I really welcomed the darkness. Believe me, the idea of not being seen was very appealing to me. My neurological confusion ran wild during the entire movie. In no time at all I had to turn away or close my eyes altogether. I simply could not keep up with any of it. The confusion was so intense.

My date knew that I had been involved in an accident, of course. Her brother and I had told her about many of my existing problems. One of the problems that I had neglected to tell her about was my spasm problem. The darkness in the movie theater didn't last long enough. I did manage to fight off my involuntary muscle spasms until we had left the show, but about halfway home it was shake, rattle, and roll time. My spasms really were mild and they never lasted much over three minutes. I didn't roll around on the ground, but they were embarrassing just the same. When these spasms did occur, my upper extremities, mainly my shoulders, would jerk around, twitch, and shake. During one of my spasm episodes, trying to speak was very difficult also.

My good friend's sister, although younger than me by at least three years, was an extremely understanding person. Unfortunately that fact was not enough for me at the time. I was in need of a lot more than understanding. I was looking for direction and needed help in finding that direction. For the young TBI survivor, help in finding even the slightest direction can be imperative.

It was a couple more bad experiences like the one I have just told you about that led me to believe that the neighborhood bar was the place for me. That's where I could go to feel sorry for myself and find plenty of company to boot. I would always find my comfort zone at the neighborhood bar. What a huge waste!

For the first ten years after the onset of my affliction, neither help nor direction was anywhere to be found. The whys of that statement are multifaceted, for certain. I'm sure I have already mentioned more than once that giving up was something that I did not know how to do. Major General Oliver P. Smith, USMC once said, "Retreat, hell! We're just attacking in another direction." With a lot of anger, and wearing my disappointment with God and life on my sleeve, attack is exactly what I did for many years. By always being on the attack, I believed I was avoiding fight or flight in a very real way. Twisted, I'm sure, but nonetheless real. My reality had become one big out-of-control act. I was headed absolutely nowhere with my recovery—not very fast at all, but extremely steadily.

Finally at the end of my rope, I had very little hope or self-esteem left. I was quite simply void, or so it seemed, of real emotion. I thought I still knew right from wrong, though I would tell you in a heartbeat that I just didn't give a damn. I'm sure I said "I don't care" one hundred times a day or more.

I was, as I have said, getting nowhere. Feeling sorry for myself was the uniform of the day. Alcohol abuse and drug misuse were not empowering me, they were robbing me and overpowering me, big time, both physically and mentally. I was one large basket case.

Finally, I made up my mind that I was going to attack in that other direction—forever, if that's what it took. My USMC experience had taught me that. But at the same time, I had to accept the fact that getting well was not part of the deal. Fortunately, I realized the best thing I could possibly do was to accept whatever life sent my way with a minimal amount of resistance. My LBO experience had taught me that. If combining the two strategies sounds contradictory to you, think about it again.

Fight or flight, either one, has seldom been appropriate for me after TBI. Although I have been faced with, from the beginning, one red light situation after another, I had determined to "attack in another direction" against any and all resistance. Attack and attack again. I was the aggressor, trying always to be in the offensive mode. How could I take flight? How could I stand and fight? I could not do either one effectively. I needed to learn to give up and not give up at the same time. Without the peace I have found in knowing my Lord and Savior Jesus Christ, I am very sure I would still be attacking in *all* directions, and I would not be sitting here today.

In a little less than a decade I found the bottom of my self-pity barrel. First I saw the bottom of the barrel and then and only then came the light—a light that I felt was strangely familiar in so many ways, I must admit. Since then, my anger has been replaced with a strong faith in Jesus Christ. I have definitely learned to relax and live. Not that I don't become angry anymore. I do. I will tell you this, though: The hate is completely gone. I still act inappropriately at times—more often than I would like to. I still suffer many effects of TBI on a daily basis.

You might be surprised to know how many people there are in this world who would choose to disbelieve the problems a TBI survivor has. I have had a difficult time believing most of what I'm telling you myself.

Many people who are living with TBI look fine at first glance. That's one of my biggest problems. I don't have any missing arms or legs. I don't have any obvious residual paralyses. However, I am, to this day, seldom if ever given the path of least resistance.

It seemed to me that my overall situation was becoming worse with the passage of time. When you look like a Porsche and run like a Volkswagen Karmann Ghia, misunderstood is what you often are. I may have been healing to some extent, but my brain cells were definitely not. All show and no go! Believe you me, I was working overtime at hiding the "no go" part of the equation.

Prior to TBI I was extremely athletic looking. Not a bad looking guy according to the standards of the day. I was also extremely active. I was a well-spoken person and one who seldom had problems with his peers. Many people had considered me to be a real man's man. After TBI, I was left with a fair resemblance of my old self. In actuality, as any real man's man of that day would tell you, I could not pour piss out of a boot. I have accepted the idea gradually over the years that telling people, up front, about my brain injury and my boot and piss problem is the best thing to do. Believe me, that's much easier for me to do as an old man than it was for me to do as a young man. At the time, for me to accept any type of limitations pertaining to what I could or could not do was absolutely impossible. I was just plain not going to do it.

I remember, very distinctly, thinking that one morning I was going to wake up and everything would be back the way it was before this horrific occurrence in my life ever took place. Battle over! Well, that never happened. I think I had gotten the idea in the first place from a doctor in Chicago. He had talked about the abnormal pressure in my brain subsiding as the contusions healed. But he was also the one who informed me of the fact that brain cells, once destroyed, do not mend or rebuild themselves, and gave me a 40-60 chance of ever walking, talking, or seeing correctly again. But if you see by sight alone in this world, you are in big trouble.

Although I never did simply wake up one morning completely healed, I did notice what I can only describe as incredible plateaus of recovery, or awakenings to recovery. These plateaus were like subtle connections being made in my brain, subtle repairs, just within reach of the outermost part of my strange state of consciousness. This always seemed to happen, when and if it indeed happened at all, only in the morning after awakening from a deep sleep.

Extreme study or concentration the day before seemed to help trigger these unusual occurrences, but not always. When this happened, I was able to say to myself with certainty, "I sure am a lot brighter today than I was yesterday." Of course, no one else ever seemed to notice. Quite strange occurrences, these awakenings, and very hard to explain to anyone, but they were welcomed. Whatever they were, they began happening after I was back in NMB. I enjoyed these plateaus or awakenings for years. To this day I continue to expect more of them. With God, all things are possible. Have I said that a couple of times already? You bet I have!

I even tried to go back to work many times. Without exception, when I would attempt to find a way to make a living I would imagine myself as the Great Imposter (the name of a movie I remembered seeing once upon a time). I would act, fake it, and try to appear as normal as possible. I always had an excuse for not filling out an application. It's amazing, but I was actually successful a couple of times. Nothing along those lines ever lasted very long, however. You can believe that any time I did get hired, the people doing the hiring were hiring almost any breathing being.

The female owner of a cab company in North Miami Beach apparently felt awfully sympathetic towards me, and she hired me as a driver. She had absolutely no idea that I was only five years post TBI. I told her I was an ex-marine. Apparently she only heard what she wanted to hear. Good. I allowed her to convince herself that I had been injured in 'Nam without saying a word. She didn't realize how bad my vision and perceptions were.

Less than ten days later it was all over. She had already had at least two negative reports concerning my driving, but I was only asked to leave after I turned my cab in one night without any door handles on the right side. My neurological neglect had gotten the best of me. I had really put up a good fight. I mean, there was hardly a scratch on either door, but they had been wiped clean of handles. The mailbox, with which I had made ever-so-slight contact, was left standing. No one could tell. I thank God every day that I never killed anyone.

Yes, sir! Any recovery was extremely slow and slight, and with each plateau I seemed to become a little more capable of getting myself into trouble. And I did, over and over again.

Unfortunately, I continue to suffer some very real effects of TBI. I deal with many psychological overlays to this very day. I also have some physical and other residual problems. Regardless, I will certainly tell you this: I have never once had to face adversity alone since I accepted Christ as my savior, and I have actually become comfortable with my neurological confusion over the years.

Comfortable with confusion might sound crazy to you. It probably should sound that way to you—but not to me. I have fought neurological confusion for years and that confusion has lost many a battle. I believe I have also been very successful in my attempts at getting other parts of my brain to take over for the damaged areas. I simply did not accomplish any of these things alone!

A couple of other things that seemed to help me quite a bit in the beginning, when I could remember to do them, of course, were silent counting and reminder notes. I counted from one to one hundred over and over again, slowly, silently and very deliberately, in, of all places, the shower. I did a lot of counting in the shower. Any cognitive improvement was so slight that the whole exercise seemed to be a big waste of time. However, the slightest reflection of the consciousness that I had known prior to TBI was more than welcomed by me. Believe me, it was not a waste of time at all for me to count in the shower. I'm still counting in the shower today. Why? I'm not really sure why. No singing! Just counting. It works for me.

As for the reminder notes, the first time someone suggested that I use notes as a way of reminding myself to do certain things that I had been forgetting to do (and believe me, I still can't remember what any of those things were), it only served to add to my discouragement. It can be a real pain trying to remind yourself of all sorts of things by using notes when you can't even remember having written them in the first place.

I thought that the idea of notes was just plain stupid. I won't say what I was thinking about the person who was offering the idea. And yes, I did sing my little one-liner at that time. Using the reminder notes did prove to be an outstanding idea. And the idea of putting a note where I was sure to find it and hopefully recognize it as something more than just another piece of paper that someone else had left lying around eventually paid off. At first, though, even after writing and finding a note that I had written for myself, I was completely lost as to its meaning, if indeed it had any.

Most people can benefit to some degree from reminder notes. In my case, though, from those undecipherable notes of mine came a vast array of different ways to bring about recall. For instance, I found that if I wrote a note just before I went to sleep and put it in an odd place like inside my shoe, I would not only find the note the next morning but also know why I had put it in there in the first place. Most of us have heard about the man who tied the string around his finger as a reminder of something and then forgot why he did that. I'm that man for sure! Learning to use a great deal of abstract thinking, learning to accept living in some strange abstract world, and dealing with your strange thoughts is not fun. That sort of thing has become my reality and for sure having fun with it has become a priority.

Like the time I waved at a friend in North Miami Beach after I had only been out of the hospital for a short time. For the life of me I could not pull my hand back down for what seemed an eternity. Finally I had to let go of my walker and risk falling in order to grab my misbehaving arm and pull it down to my side.

Or how about the time, years later, when I was out selling accident insurance, trying hard to do that, anyway, and I knocked on someone's front door only to forget, completely, what it was I was doing there in the first place. By the time the person came to the door, my mind apparently went blank. That was not the first time I had experienced this type of thing, so I knew just what to do. Before leaving that front door I had a real good laugh and sold some insurance as well.

Nowadays if I ring your doorbell and I can't remember why, I'll simply tell you a detailed story about some fantastic something or other until the real reason I'm there comes to me. If I happen to be selling something, you'll more than likely buy one or two of them, anyway.

If you're wondering how I ever got a license to sell insurance, join the club! I wonder about that myself. All of my attempts at selling anything came after I had successfully completed my training for the Baptist ministry and my rote memory was working exceptionally well...when it was working. I took a State of Florida insurance test and I passed it. At that time my full scale I.Q. was a sporadic 137 or better. Not bad at all for a guy with TBI. In February of 1965 I had a full-scale I.Q. of 93 without much hope for improvement.

I was told that I would never walk, talk, or see correctly again, but that certainly was not going to be the last word as far as I was concerned. Not in my world. Believe you me, the operative word in the above statement has always been the word *correctly*. Not being able to do something correctly doesn't mean that you can't do it at all. By attempting, over and over again, to do all of the things that I could no longer do, my ability to concentrate was reaching a new high. But getting other people to understand and accept that fact has never been easy. Getting others to accept me as a productive and worthwhile human being has been my biggest challenge. After all, at age sixty-two I still have a real problem saying my ABC's, and multiplication tables are impossible for me. That's not an easy thing for a man who accomplished a 3.7 overall GPA in college to say, or to accept, for that matter.

I did finally come up with enough right answers to earn a bachelor's degree and to claim back most of my awareness. Like I have already said, it's tough for anyone to argue with success. I am and have been very aware of almost everything for some time now. I think so, anyway. Until recently some normal folks were still trying to question my behavior. I can only hope that they have all given up by now.

I would like to share parts of my earliest psychological evaluation with you. This evaluation was done on February 22, 1965 at the request of Vocational Rehabilitation of the State of Florida, approximately 17 months after my accident. My reason for including this document is the sincere hope that you will gain more understanding about TBI in terms of recovery. But remember: No two cases of TBI are exactly alike.

Psychological Examination of Blakemore, Joseph T.

Mr. Blakemore was referred for psychological examination by his VR counselor in conjunction with his evaluation for vocational rehabilitation. Mr. Blakemore was in a serious automobile accident on Aug. 30, 1963, which apparently left him with a problem of balance and some speech difficulty. There is a distinct slurring of speech and Mr. Blakemore's description of the difficulty that he has in groping for words strongly suggests a mild expressive aphasia.

At the present time, he is totally uncertain about what he wants to do, but under pressure admits that he would like to be an actor or in some field of the dramatics. Mr. Blakemore is interested in going back to school.

He had considerable difficulty initially in finding the examiner's office and was late for his first appointment. It was necessary to schedule a second appointment. He was quite reluctant to use a pencil and paper and under some duress did complete the Bender and Drawings. After he had left the examiner's office, he called the examiner, indicating that he did not want the results of this first set of drawings included at all and that he would like to try to do them again, to see if he could do better. It took considerable reassurance to convince him that this would not be necessary, that the examiner had taken into consideration the fact that Mr. Blakemore had not used a pencil and paper in some time.

While anxious about his production and about what he should do, he had difficulty in improving his performance. He was most uncertain about his future and obviously depressed and upset by it, in spite of the fact that his tension outlet seems to be lacking, rather than a more appropriate kind of affect in view of the serious limitations that have been imposed on him since his accident. The more tense he became, the more labile laughter was noted and the more the examiner felt that this was grossly inappropriate considering the way the man obviously felt.

It seems evident that this man was of at least above average intellectual potential, but this potential has been reduced to an average to low average level. Thus, on the Wechsler he obtains the following I.Q. estimates:

Verbal I.Q.: 96
Performance I.Q.: 92
Full Scale I.Q.: 93

Qualitatively, reasoning tends to be quite concrete and there is relatively poor control over impulsive behavior. Abstract reasoning is impaired to the point where it would be difficult for this man to function in a higher academic setting and when confronted with relatively unfamiliar and/or complicated situations, he tends to become rather disorganized and, as mentioned above, labile.

There is enormous underlying depression and as he grows older and less able, from a realistic standpoint, to function competitively, it is felt that the danger of suicidal attempts will increase. The impairment of various psychological processes and of emotional control is felt to be severe and probably permanent. This great a relative reduction in intellectual functioning and learning capacity is seriously incapacitating to the personality.

It seems evident that Mr. Blakemore has really not arrived at any successful adjustment or acceptance of his limitations. He is in need of counseling and probably should be under the care of a physician, preferably a psychiatrist, to help handle the turmoil that he experiences and perhaps to assist him to view his limitations more realistically. It is felt that he can function to about 75% of efficiency in semi-skilled tasks such as production and assembly work, but his self-concept and needs will make it very difficult for him to accept this kind of a come-down in aspirations. It is highly unlikely that there will be any major change, if the accident did indeed happen in 1963. Ideally, it is felt that this man would be able to function best in a protective or semi-sheltered training situation, but getting him to accept this will be a serious problem. Generally, prognosis for successful emotional and competitive adjustment is only fair.

The Ph.D. who administered my first psychological examination in 1965 suggested training in a sheltered setting. In my case, endeavoring to become a professional student worked surprisingly well. In spite of my disease I was still able to learn. I could learn how to do something one day and not know how to do that same thing the very next day. My ability to learn it over again, however, was constant.

Testing my I.Q. today is problematic for sure, and probably will remain that way. I, on the other hand, have been more than happy to accept the findings of the last attempt. The last psychological evaluation was done by the Veterans Administration in 1976. On that day my full-scale I.Q. was 137. That was quite a few years before completing my undergraduate studies, also. I have absolutely no idea what my I. Q. is at this time. I really don't have much concern in that area any longer. Anything over full-scale 93 looks really good to me, and 137 and over makes me very happy.

Once again, I'm not blowing my own horn. I did it and you can, too. Even if you never get as far as I have (I'm not at all sure how far that is, after all. Once brain damaged, always brain damaged), just bear in mind that I never did get as far as some other folks, either. The personal understanding that we gain while attempting to overcome some of life's problems by giving them our best shot is very rewarding. The idea of never allowing oneself to fall victim to self-pity has proven to be paramount, and at the same time my accident proved to be a true blessing.

Most everything I have done since my accident in 1963, with few exceptions, has been like doing whatever it is for the very first time. That's just the reality of my TBI, and I readily accept it today. I knew that retention was not the problem in my case. Of course, convincing anyone else of that was difficult. I knew from the beginning that everything I was taking in was remaining somewhere in my damaged brain. I never knew when something I had learned was going to emerge, or how much of it for that matter. Trying to get a handle on the workings of my damaged brain has been unbelievably interesting. The idea of being a lifetime student worked well, I believe, because my rote memory is the one part of my memory that is closest to being normal. I have long since given up on the idea of my brain healing. To some extent, though, other parts of my brain have taken over for the dead or damaged brain cells. My brain will never be the same. I will never be the same. Believe me, I'm all the better for it.

The single greatest benefit to me, other than something supernatural in my life, has been the sheer mechanics of higher education. Knowing you know so much about so many different things, and at the same time not being able to use that knowledge or communicate it to others, can be extremely frustrating to say the least. But with the Lord's help all things are possible and the accomplishments of any human being can be endless. I'm sixty-two years young and I'm just getting started!

I have always tried to do the things that people said I would never do again. Running was one of those things, and walking was another. Running has proven to be impossible for me, forever and for sure. As far as my walking is concerned, I no longer walk like I once did, and I still fall and bump into things sometimes.

Many people who suffer TBI find that their memory, both short-term and long-term, has agendas all of its own. Shoot! My entire brain has had, at the very least, some strange and odd memories, no doubt. I knew that I had learned how to do many things prior to TBI. Being told about these things, and having my recall slowly and sporadically return only added to the dilemma when so much of the physical wouldn't respond at all.

Nonetheless, I was determined to learn more than I had known at the time of my accident. I figured that no matter how much I knew at any given time, I needed to know more. I'm not at all certain that knowledge was the complete answer to my memory situation. In fact, I'm certain that it wasn't. But having more resources to draw from hasn't hurt me one bit.

Although it took me much too long to learn, I finally did approximately ten years later. I learned what satire was all about. Satire and the ability to laugh at ourselves is one of the greatest gifts God has ever given any of us. Try it, you'll like it! Today I make it a point to laugh at myself often. I'm not going to try and tell you that I have been laughing ever since. I still find myself in my darn fish bowl every once in a while. But through it all, my laughing is still very much intact. Satire has often been a fantastic pop-off valve for me.

I have this strange desire to tell the world just how much I have enjoyed the ringing of my bell, but in reality we all know a statement like that is simply not correct. Then again there might just be a lot to be said for people who put the square pegs in round holes and become successful at it. The point I'm trying to make here is one that has been made before. I'm okay and so are you.

Believe me, I knew from the beginning that I had potential and I was convinced that I could improve. I became all the more convinced with even the slightest improvement in my condition. This was always the case even when other people appeared to be much less impressed with me. So what? Understanding a particular concept and yet not being able to complete a single task required in the proving of that concept can be frustrating and empowering simultaneously. Welcome to TBI 101. Like I said earlier, one must learn to have fun with drain bamage!

My unspoken motto for the most part has always been "If at first you don't succeed, try, try again." The people who have helped me most since my accident have been the people in my life who have allowed me to do just that: try again and again and again and then again. If you are a TBI survivor, or the family member of a TBI survivor, or the significant other of a TBI survivor, the sooner you both understand that you will always be trying again, the easier your life will become. I could not have done that by myself.

The psychologist said, "It is highly unlikely that there will be any major change." Don't you just love it? My experience has taught me one big bunch of lessons—way more than I can count. I'll have TBI forever. It's my baggage forever. But I am more than a little bit pleased to be able to say that today I am walking, talking, and seeing fairly well. Of course, old age is beginning to do its thing. Be that as it may, I have still come a long, long way. I have had to learn to accept the fact that everything is constantly changing, and, in many cases, remains different and difficult. That almost sounds normal, doesn't it?

CHAPTER 8

God's Grace and Graceville

After my discharge from Elmhurst General Hospital in 1963, everything seemed to be moving at the speed of light—except for me, of course. I was unbelievably slow, both mentally and physically. There was apparently no place and no one for me to turn to for help at that time.

My mother told me sometime after I found myself back in Miami that there were simply not any affordable rehabilitation programs available to me. As a matter of fact, it was specifically written on my medical chart form Elmhurst General Hospital that I was not recommended for rehabilitation. Give me a break. Not recommended for rehabilitation, at any cost?

My mother's assumption was probably correct. Even if we had had a lot of money, knowing where to get help with my problem in that day and age was tough. Still, I'd like to think we would have at least given it our best shot, money obstacles or not. But that's wishful thinking on my part. My stepfather, like many other folks at that time, did not believe in insurance much at all. He had never carried health or accident insurance on my sister or me.

Even if there had been rehabilitation programs available for TBI victims at that time, my folks were not about to find a dime (or the time, either) for anything like that. The situation I was in was definitely not a priority for them. Things may have been different if I had not been so rebellious as a teen. My situation was my responsibility, and the sooner I came to grips with that fact, the better.

I was a twenty-two-year-old adult at the time of my accident. I should have had my own coverage, and I would have if I had been with International Harvester long enough. As a matter of fact, I did have *some* coverage with them. Talk about fate. Just forty-five minutes prior to my accident, my hospitalization coverage went into force. Ma and Pa, the Engstroms, were ready to mortgage their home on my behalf when they got the good news: My extended stay in the hospital was completely paid for by insurance.

My mother actually did take me to see our family doctor once—the same doctor who had delivered my younger half sister Karen in 1956. His office was located not too far from where we lived at the time.

All the family doctor could say was that I was "way too fancy for him." I never did forget that. I was way too fancy. I guess I've been way too fancy for quite a while now. He suggested that they take me to the neurology department at Jackson Memorial Hospital in Miami. Fancy, Fancy, Fancy. I can tell you for certain that the folks at Jackson did not know that much about my brain injury, either, but to my surprise an appointment with Dr. Peritz Scheinberg, a world-renowned neurologist, was made.

The visit to Jackson Memorial had both a positive and negative impact on my recovery attempts. Dr. Scheinberg told me that there wasn't a person in the world who knew what I was faced with or could fix or repair my damaged brain. The doctor went on to say that my chance for a full recovery was non-existent. Medical science had not gathered half of the information about the human brain and its functions that it has today, and it continues to have a long way to go in its absolute understanding thereof. I had to accept my fate as being permanent.

It was at that point that I felt the strength of his gaze as his eyes fixed directly on mine. For the first time in my life, I felt like I was in the presence of a truly superior human being. I was trying with all of my being to understand his every word. At that moment, though, I was struggling to retain one word after another. Everything he said seemed to flash in and flash out, and I had no time at all for inductive or deductive reasoning. But somehow, through it all, I knew I had gotten every word, even if I did lack the ability to repeat any of it.

In a soft yet extremely firm tone he asked, "Joseph, are you a man of faith?" Feeling a very strange and almost desperate need to answer yes, I stammered. He shifted his gaze toward my mother. "I am a devout Jew," he said. "In the Torah—you call it the Old Testament of the Bible—I have found a verse that speaks of unplowed ground. I'm not going to attempt to tell you about my faith, but I want you to remember this: We all have a great deal of unplowed ground up here." He pointed to his head. "We don't know that much about it. Joseph, I believe that it's possible for you to train the unused portion of your brain, the 'unplowed ground,' so to speak, to take over for the damaged areas. You must understand that it is all up to you and your creator." Looking at my mother once more, he smiled, tilted his head and said, "I'm sorry. There is nothing else I can say."

Somehow what Dr. Scheinberg said was recorded and stored in my damaged cerebellum. I have been able to draw strength from his words many times since then. I was awake and alive, sitting in a chair in his office, but I was in a state of consciousness that I had certainly never experienced before TBI. Popeye, Spinach, and the Holy Bible kept running through my head. "You am what you am, and that's all you am, kid!" That was the first thing my mother said to me in the car on the way home. I remember that warm, all-knowing smile. I think.

Apparently, what my mother took with her from our meeting with Dr. Scheinberg was somewhat different than what I came away with. My mother would remain extremely skeptical about any type of recovery on my part. Others questioned my memory and retention capability, and I found myself going along with whatever was said even when I knew better. I can't really explain how it was or how it is. Awkward. Very awkward. A person has to experience TBI in order to really believe or understand any of it, in my opinion. I think it might be important for you to know (especially if you deal with people who have experienced TBI) that I was retaining everything. Recall was and still is sporadic at best, even with my long- and short-term memories seemingly improving over the years (emphasis on "seemingly"). I'm certain that I do remember sitting there in Dr. Scheinberg's office, though, struggling to grasp every word. It's like I said, I was in a state of consciousness that I had not known before, and being told that I was going to have to do my best with it...what did it all mean? I know for sure that I felt as though this event was quite a privilege. The motivation that I have found in that doctor's words has been priceless. It was indeed a privilege for my mother and me to have the opportunity to talk to this man. My God, his God, the creator of mankind has become manifest in my life a countless number of times since that day in 1964. The only answer is indeed God.

From the very first day after having been flown back to "nothing, NMB" and the home of my mother and stepfather, my main objective was to get out of there somehow—anyhow! Escape! I guess I always knew that the only way to accomplish that was for me to get better, but how was I going to get better without some sort of a structured program aimed at overcoming all of my neurological problems? I mean, there I was, far from being in a total state of vegetation, and yet, on the other hand, a long, long way from being a normal person. Mr. In-between can make a fellow mean, for sure. What to do about it became my repeated question. "What am I and what can I possibly become?" The doctors I had seen since the day of my misfortune had all told me the same thing: "We don't know enough about your brain at this time to be of much help."

Vocational Rehabilitation of the State of Florida did not have a single answer for me in 1964. (DVR has always been a bit on the shortsighted side of things.) The idea that I had become totally unemployable, and that no one at that time seemed to be interested in thinking in long-term scenarios when it came to my case, was very frustrating. What was even more frustrating was the fact that I had lost much of my ability to communicate my frustration without losing my cool altogether.

It seemed like trouble followed me about constantly and I could not tolerate my frustration at all. The only limitation I was willing to accept was something that I knew to be absolute. For instance, in my case, I knew I would never run again. I also knew that there were many things I could do or might do in time. If no one wanted to give me a break, then I would take matters in my own hands. So, swallowed up in self-pity and with a devil-may-care attitude, the highway was soon to become my way. I was simply not going to do things their way and it didn't matter who they were, either. The drummer to whose beat I was marching was very different indeed—strange more often than not. Like I told you earlier, nothing was there. There appeared to be absolutely nothing available for any TBI survivors in 1963. "You am what you am, kid!" Believe me, that's all any of us can be.

Moving in my newfound direction, I was determined to make my own breaks, good or bad. (Don't just stand there! Do something! Even if it's wrong!) I'm not at all sure of what was going on with my thinking at the time. Other than the consistent thought that my life was hell on earth, I'm not sure that I was thinking at all. Reality as I had come to know it prior to TBI was gone, and I was being told that this was a permanent state. My only reality (when I was cognizant enough to realize it) was sink or swim, live or die. The odds? Not in my favor.

I guess I figured that even if I had to do everything the hard way, walking, talking, seeing, etc., I'd rather attempt to do that than listen to all of the people telling me what I could not do—could never do. That sort of talk just led to more depression. I was just plain sick. The sooner I could get out from under the thumbs of all of the nay-sayers, the better.

Living with TBI was something that I simply did not want to do any longer. As far as I was concerned, I had become one of life's biggest losers. There wasn't anything worth living for. To put it in the vernacular of today, everything sucked! There was no one for me to turn to and I really didn't give a rat's butt about anything or anyone.

The first nine years or so of my ordeal were awful and extremely awkward. Energy seemed to come back to me very slowly. At first, all I wanted to do was sleep. Then, after a year or more, all I wanted to do was learn to walk and, at the same time, successfully hide the fact that I was about to fall flat on my face.

I have had to learn to use my athletic ability to compensate for my physical problems. It was as though my brain was disconnected from my body more often than not. Exactly how I managed to stay alive, let alone improve at all in my condition, is hard to figure. All I can tell you is that I never stopped trying, and with God's help, my energy finally did return in abundance.

So, with $40 in my pocket, I headed for the Sunshine State Parkway, or Florida's Turnpike, drain bamage and all. Look out world! If you're questioning the "and all" part of the preceding sentence, pot, alcohol and amphetamines were all present in my bloodstream at the time. In some strange way, altering my state of consciousness during my first ten years of life with TBI always seemed to bring me closer to reality. I'm not saying that what I was doing with drugs and alcohol was the right thing to do. I'm sure it was not. But at least when someone said, "Hey, man, you're really screwed up," there was no doubt in my mind.

They were definitely referring to a reality of some kind. I try hard not to use TBI as an excuse for any of my bad behavior, but you have to admit it is a good one, at that. Of course, if you use something, anything, as a constant excuse for not overcoming life's hardships, the chances are you will never overcome them.

After the first couple of days on the road, using a stick for a cane came so naturally that I wondered why I hadn't used one before. My double vision caused me to close one eye more than I had ever done before. I soon found out, also, that the more and the farther I walked, the easier it was to walk. I even tried to get some kind of a rhythm going with my awkward gait. (I have never lost my awkward gait but I have been very successful in deciding not to let the way I walk bother me!)

Hitchhiking is definitely not the safest way for anyone to travel. The experiences I have had out there on the road have taught me one thing for sure: Hitchhiking is for the birds! I'm not in any hurry to get back out there again. Not like that, anyway.

Hitching rides around the United States in my condition was certainly not the best or the brightest thing for me to be doing, but self-pity was having its way. The overall scenario seemed to be somewhat familiar. In fact, it appeared to be the same old same old. "When you got nothing, you got nothing to lose." As I saw it, life for me was hell and I had been left with less than nothing. Please, God, tell me what kind of second chance at life this is? I have always believed in God. Maybe by heading toward the turnpike and the open highway, I felt as though I were putting God to the test. After all, he had given me a second chance at life. Why? I had truly become another homeless person. Of course, back then, people like me were simply referred to as bums or derelicts, and so I was.

Late one afternoon, I was attempting to leave the Tampa, Florida area with an ominous-looking black and blue sky peering over my favorite shoulder. I resigned myself to the fact that, like many times before, I was about to become one soggy homeless guy. I had successfully blocked out, for that moment, anyway, the fact that I had irreversible and residual brain damage. (No one I knew called brain damage TBI back then.) I was moving on down the road with my extremely awkward yet rhythmic gait. Every once in a while I heard a voice in my head calling out a marching cadence, and I could smell the incoming rain as it moved closer. The only good thing about getting wet while trying to get a free ride in Florida is that the weather, for the most part, is warm or hot, making drying out a little easier and the threat of pneumonia much less significant. I really didn't mind the rain at all. I actually liked the rain most of the time. It always seemed to make getting a ride a lot harder, though. My double vision and balance also became harder to deal with in a downpour.

With my attitude toward life at that time admittedly incorrect at best (I just didn't care!), I looked at everything in life as if it were a challenge, and it was. Everything was truly challenging, from interacting with others to communicating with myself. Walking, seeing, talking—all could be done, but the degree of difficulty that accompanied everything was indeed challenging.

Anyway, if you are familiar at all with the Tampa Bay area, you're more than likely aware of all of the bridges as well. Trying to tell you about the bridges that existed there on that bay over twenty-five years ago is a bit tricky. Everything has changed so much. I'm not at all sure what highway I was on that day, either. Even if I knew, it's bound to have a different name and/or number today. But I can tell you this firsthand: The Tampa Bay bridges of 1967 were not made for people to walk on, especially people suffering from TBI.

The next thing that I was absolutely fully aware of was that the rain was coming down, seemingly sideways and in buckets. I had made it halfway across one of those extremely low-lying bay bridges—bridges that sit right down on top of the shark-infested water. How or why, I haven't the first clue. Not the how or why of the bridge or the water or the shark infestation, but how or why I was, of all places, in the middle of them with TBI.

I have thought about that day in '67 many times over the years. I just can't figure it all out. I draw a blank. I think I got into a car at a traffic light, and that's it. I can't figure it out. If I could tell you more I would, believe you me.

All I could do was pray and try not to look at the water if I wanted to maintain my balance. My balance was my priority. The motion of the water with its brightly dancing little whitecaps was dizzying enough. Neuro-confusion seemed to wrap tightly around my head. Perception of anything was hard to hang on to. Now add to the whole scenario, if you will, the semi trucks flying by at sixty miles an hour or better and some cars as well, all of which would be followed by wind and rain. Well, if you are me, you figure yourself to be one dead duck—a soggy, homeless dead duck. Dead! Oh well. My "I don't care" attitude remained intact, and I was calm and deliberate throughout my little ordeal. I questioned my lack of emotion. I didn't think I would get off that bridge alive. Where was my fear of dying? Where, my urgent reaction to being in harm's way? A battle was occurring, big time, between my physical and mental being and a soul that simply had to live. Although I really didn't care, at least consciously, about living and I seemed not to have any fear of death, something definitely kept me from offering any help at all to the Grim Reaper that night. I didn't know why at the time, but I'm sure I know now. Every time I look into my wife's eyes or into the eyes of my son or daughter, say hello to one of our dogs or cats, touch a leaf, or see the sky, I know!

On either side of one of those Tampa Bay bridges, there was a narrow place to accommodate the walking of a normal person. However, those were only to be used in an emergency, and ideally only after all traffic on the bridge had been halted. The trucks that flew by were so close to me that I know I felt at least one of them brush my shirtsleeve. I'm tempted to believe that at least one of the drivers of those big trucks made a deliberate attempt to bump me off. Of course, the wind and rain that followed a single truck were enough to blow anyone off a bridge of that type.

Suddenly I realized that I was teetering back and forth, standing and barely balancing on one leg. A vision of all the sharks swimming around beneath those small whitecaps became crystal clear in my mind's eye. What took place next was amazing and dumbfounding as well. I don't recall moving beyond the middle of that bridge after the rain began falling. The portion of the bridge that I find myself doing my balancing act on was the end—the east end of the bridge. My mind did not readily accept this fact. I felt my body pivoting around on my right foot, and my left leg was lifted in preparation to dismount my peril.

How did I get to the end of the bridge? Why did I get to the end of the bridge? My reality and a somewhat clearer perception came back to me with a jolt as my weak left knee buckled only slightly and managed to absorb and hold my full body weight. I was clear of the bridge, dazed and trying very hard to understand what had just happened to me. I was surprised once again that the rain was completely gone and the early evening Tampa Bay sky was clear as could be. A car slid deliberately off the pavement and onto the lightly graveled shoulder of the road. It came to a full and abrupt stop about forty yards ahead of me. I was still pretty much out of it. Everything would be fine with me if I could just get back to my fish bowl!

The awareness I had of the car became all the more manifest to me when the driver, a man who appeared to be in his early to mid thirties, came running towards me, shouting, "What the hell are you trying to do, man? Kill yourself, or what?"

"I guess I need a ride!" Those words just kind of fell out of my mouth with a bit more slur than usual.

"I guess you do! How in the hell did you get out here, anyways?"

As we got into his car, his questions kept coming and I could feel myself slipping back into my fish bowl. Little did the guy know, but I was absolutely unable to answer any of his questions. I did mutter something about my brain damage and confusion. I don't believe he got any of it. He went on talking. He may well have been talking even after I passed out or went to sleep. Oh well! Like my son would say today, whatever!

When I woke up, we were in Gainesville, Florida and the man was still talking. He was still rattling on when I thanked him for the ride and closed his car door. I don't think I'll ever forget the last thing old motor mouth had to say as his car door was being closed: "I think God is trying to tell you something, boy."

I'm quite certain that divine intervention saved me from certain death that night. No doubt about it.

But it was not until I found myself at the end of my rope, the bottom of the barrel, and believed the world and I would be much better off if I never saw the light of another day, that I finally saw the true light. I made a public profession of my faith in 1970 in the First Baptist Church of Greater Miami, almost nine years after sustaining TBI. God's grace is truly amazing.

I often wonder if anyone else in this world has had the same type of in-depth conversations with himself that I have had. Something tells me that there is more than one of us out here. Few of us older folks have made it this far in life without someone telling us how bad it is to talk to oneself. I never did believe that, and besides, I really enjoy talking to a good person every so often. Because I'm a TBI survivor, the ability to talk to myself, and to answer also, has proven to be a real blessing. It goes without saying that having the right answers to many of my own questions has been a big plus, but that certainly has not always been the case.

Take my question as to why I had been given a second chance to begin with. I am convinced and absolutely certain that I know the answer to that question today. However, at that time, if I knew the answer to that question, I was not about to admit that to anyone—myself included. Furthering my education was my only interest, and that appeared to be a dead-end street for some very obvious reasons. The opportunity for me to advance my level of education came my way only after my acceptance of Christ in 1970. Oddly enough, then and only then did the doors to higher education begin opening for me. It is my belief that had I not experienced the grace of God in the way that I did in Graceville, my story could never have had a just and happy ending. Christ has been the answer in my life.

In 1971, I began studying at Baptist Bible Institute, BBI, or as it is called today, BCF, Baptist College of Florida, which is located in a very small town in north Florida called Graceville— a very appropriate name, indeed. The sheer grace I received from God in that small town, located right smack in what some folks call the Bible belt, is extremely hard to understand or to explain. However, without the grace of God, I'm quite sure I would have never finished my coursework there and I would definitely not be the person I am today. I spent four of the best, most worthwhile, and what I consider to have been miraculous years of my life there.

I know beyond a shadow of a doubt that God called me to BBI to study in preparation for his will in my life, but I had to bring my "born again" energy into the classroom and allow my mind to be challenged extensively. God has allowed me to use some unplowed ground—parts of my brain that I had never used prior to my auto accident in 1963. I could have never learned to compensate as well as I have, physically or mentally, without this re-channeling of energy and the God-given ability to train other parts of my brain to compensate for the damaged portions.

I had been learning all along how to deal with a host of neurological deficits. My eyesight was absolutely inexplicable. Reading textbooks and the Bible with one eye closed in order to compensate for my diplopia (double vision) was simply one of the many awkward things I had to resign myself to. "Compensate" should, more than likely, be my middle name. If you have experienced TBI, and if you are aware of yourself and your surroundings to any acceptable degree, I'm sure you can identify with compensating, and it could probably be your middle name, too. One thing I certainly can attest to: Simply becoming acutely aware of a problem—physical, mental, or combined—is truly half of the battle. In my opinion, what I have just told you is physiologically sound, although I am certainly not an expert in physiology. In short, the more you know about all of your parts and their relationships, one to another (in the context of what I like to think of as the Devine trichotomy: mind, body, and spirit), the better off your whole being becomes.

As an example, the more I learned about my brain in the context of mind, body, and spirit, the more readily the paralysis of the left side of my body seemed to subside. (Today, any residual paralysis is very subtle.) This faith-based philosophy, I like to call it my applied philosophy, seemed to be applicable to all of my neurological problems, from memory loss to emotional control problems, and a host of others as well.

At BBI, the understanding of my brain damage by both faculty and students was poor at best. I really did feel as though everyone there, at one time or another, had misunderstood me. From the beginning, I admittedly skirted the issues pertaining to my health. A close friend advised me not to mention my head injury at all, and I didn't. So it was no real surprise to me that there wasn't much understanding about my brain damage. I never told them. By my third, and what should have been the last, year of my enrollment, I'm sure the word was out. Although I was never confronted with my brain damage issues while at BBI, it's unthinkable that the faculty there did not figure it all out. My behavior was questionable from time to time. But I was very sure of God's love and understanding in my life, and the *overall* understanding and acceptance I received while studying at BBI was God-sent, I'm certain!

I had been somewhat successful at my attempts to isolate myself from all but a select group of people during the time I spent there. God-fearing people surrounded me, and in my opinion God-fearing people are the very best people. Isolation is certainly not the key to overcoming TBI. I more than realize that every case is extraordinarily different. However, in my case, isolation, the passage of time, the sheer mechanics of higher education, and faith in the Lord Jesus Christ had proven extremely advantageous over that four-year period. My faith, my education and patient, prayerful, persistent perseverance would prove to be extremely advantageous to me throughout my entire life. It is very hard to argue with success, and it is impossible for anyone to take your education away from you. Education and faith—what a combination. It works for me!

Let me assure you, there is absolutely no end in sight to my compensating, both physically and mentally. Having patience is not easy, either. At least for me, it isn't. You must go on, winning battle after battle, while fully understanding that you will never win the war—in the temporal sense, that is. The silver lining here, for me anyway, was that God created man to be the most adaptable organism in all creation. I read that in a contemporary psychology and effective behavior textbook one day, and I have done my best to keep it in the forefront of my mind ever since. The USMC had taught me field expedience. Now this was a whole new ball game, for sure. Compensate! Compensate! Compensate! Adapt! Adapt! Adapt!

I was licensed to preach in 1972, and I did have the opportunity to preach a number of times. I even gave the eulogy at my stepfather's funeral in 1974. My stepfather, having spent some time in India during the Second World War, professed to be a Buddhist. Standing behind the pulpit on that day, I said something I simply did not intend to say. "My stepfather is going to heaven as sure as I am." Where that came from, I haven't the slightest idea. Well, maybe I do have some idea. Only a Southern Baptist preacher with brain damage would say something like that.

It took me four long years to complete a three-year curriculum at Baptist Bible Institute. In 1975, I became the recipient of a fully accredited, three-year diploma in theology.

"Rooty toot toot, rooty toot toot. We are the boys from the institute. We don't smoke. We don't chew. We don't date the girls that do. We're a bunch of sissies." Every time the word "institute" runs through my mind, it's always followed by that rhythmic, mischievous little jingle.

I don't really know why I never became a Southern Baptist pastor, took a church, or became ordained, but those doors were simply not opening for me at the time. Misspent youth? Most of the Southern Baptist churches and pulpit committees I was coming into contact with in late 1975 and '76 seemed to be looking for a married man, preferably one whose wife could play the piano. (I must admit I forgot to ask my wife if she knew how to play a piano when I asked her to marry me in '77. I did, however, ask her if she had accepted Christ as her Savior before I asked her to marry me. She said yes to both questions, and the rest is history.)

I made contact with the Southern Baptist Convention in Leon County, Florida in 1976, approximately one year after graduating from BBI (and approximately one year before my wife said yes). The associational missionary told me what I had already figured out for myself: It was very hard, next to impossible, for a single man to find a church to pastor in the Southern Baptist Convention. The fact that the nation was in a deep recession didn't help much, either. My brain damage was not cited as a roadblock, but I did mention it more than once, and I'm sure we both knew that TBI was playing a negative role in my attempts at finding a church to pastor.

But I really do think that if God had given me a wife at that time, I would have had a much better chance of finding a church to pastor. I have even entertained the idea, more than once, that if God had only given me a wife and a piano, I could have set the evangelistic world on fire. He didn't. I didn't. If the Lord wanted me to go out and pastor a church, that's exactly where I would have gone. He didn't want, so I didn't go!

My recovery has been all about faith, education, and a conscious effort to re-channel my energy. It has taken one very strong bond with the Great Physician for me to experience inner peace, the peace it takes to simply relax and overcome the prolonged and repeated stress caused by TBI.

Learning to let the Lord lead the way in my life has not been easy. I have dropped the ball many times. The storm is still raging and adversity is everywhere. However, I know I have found a safe harbor forever.

CHAPTER 9

The System? What System?

By the time I graduated from Baptist Bible Institute in 1975, my self-esteem had risen like the Apollo 11 mission that had put Armstrong, Collins, and Aldrin on the moon in July of 1969. Education and faith had become my vehicle to the stars. I could both feel and see evidence of the dramatic changes taking place in my damaged brain. Improving the quality of my life was possible—it was happening. What I was experiencing was fantastic, inexplicable, and unbelievable. I was positive at that time in my life that even if I never found a way to go back to school again, I had already managed to learn enough from some very brilliant and well-educated men at BBI to keep me headed in the right direction for all eternity. The sheer mechanics of higher education had worked wonders for me. I wanted to keep studying forever. Even today, at the age of sixty-two, my thirst for knowledge is still unquenched. But at the time, accomplishing that goal was my big dilemma. Allowing myself to become somewhat caught up in the human condition once more, I desperately tried to get help from the Department of Vocational Rehabilitation in 1976. If the rest of this chapter sounds repetitious, redundant and ridiculous, then you may have gotten my point.

This extremely difficult VR counselor got, as she put it, "stuck with my case." She refused to give any consideration to my past accomplishments. She refused to contact BBI on my behalf. As far as she was concerned, BBI was just a Bible school. She never looked into the accreditation of the school, or made any attempt to get my transcripts. Why that was not done is anyone's guess. Ultimately, my new counselor made the decision to send me to the Easter Seals job skills evaluation program. My first reaction upon hearing her decision was total shock. Then the philosophic doctrine of C. S. Peirce, Pragmatics, came to my weary mind. What was the most practical thing for me to do in this situation?

I was absolutely certain that this young lady simply did not know the first thing about brain damage. It seemed highly unlikely that she knew where to go for help with my situation either. She did, however, become awfully convincing when she explained to me that VR would continue helping me pay rent during this so-called evaluation. It was my understanding from dealing with "the system" earlier on that taking whatever they gave me was better than winding up with nothing at all.

My first attempt at getting help with my neurological problems from the State of Florida had taken place in Miami back in 1964. The people working in the Miami office at that time tried to discourage and dissuade me in every way they possibly could. Ultimately they were very successful in convincing me that rehabilitation in my case was not feasible. That was perhaps the biggest lie that anyone ever told me. I did not have much formal education at the time, and my faith was inconsistent at best. However, even in that day and age, I'm sure V R could have and should have done more. They did nothing and I wound up with nothing.

When my wife and I married in 1977, she had her state job. I was in the Easter Seals program having my job skills evaluated. The group I soon found myself a member of consisted solely of people suffering from mental retardation. This was hard for me to understand or to accept, but I forced myself to do just that. I was not about to confront VR over anything. That was not the practical thing to do. No way! Newly wed and almost penniless, I was determined to take whatever VR gave me and use it to my

advantage. Being agreeable and following their instructions to
the letter seemed to be the thing to do. Vocational Rehabilitation
was paying my rent. In exchange, all I had to do was allow them
to assign me to a group of mentally retarded folks. It wasn't
exactly the type of education I had in mind and it wasn't exactly
the type of mind I actually had, either.

I felt very awkward not having a job, and at the same time I
was growing considerably impatient waiting for divine
intervention. However, my faith was a lot more consistent then
than it had been in 1964, and I had been formally educated in the
interim as well—both big plusses. My entire situation, at least all
that I was capable of being aware of at that time, was cruelly
embarrassing and extremely hard for me to accept. Patience is a
virtue—one that I have had to work extraordinarily hard to obtain
since suffering from TBI.

Unfortunately, and on top of everything else at that time, I
seemed to be the only one, at least in my world, who was aware
of what my affliction was doing to me. I believe that my faith in
God allowed me to deal with, and overcome to a great degree,
my need for professional help—a kind of help I was not getting
from VR or anyone else.

Please don't think for one minute that I failed to realize how
much professional help I had already received in my attempt to
become educated. I will always be truly grateful for it. Reading,
writing, and recitation had been good for this TBI survivor. I
tried to get VR to send me back to school for that very reason.
Unfortunately, VR seemed content with simply sending me for
some type of evaluation every time I turned around—one dead
end after another.

I vaguely remember one man that VR had sent me to see in
1978. This particular fellow almost gave me a chance at real
employment. He was somewhat aware of my education,
experience, and my faith as well. In fact, he said he admired my

faith a great deal. I told him that if he would simply take the time to hear what it was I was trying to say, and give me a chance, I would prove myself to be a very hard-working and devoted employee. I was, I felt, certainly capable of adding to the overall success of his company. But in the end, he simply did not hear me. The man was too busy telling me about his own faith. He missed it. He didn't take the time to listen.

It has been my experience that there are far too many people in this world who don't have any idea how powerful the listening ear can actually be. Of course, the all-too-common belief that anyone who has suffered brain damage is an extremely dangerous person was evident in what he had to say as well. The man admired my faith, but nevertheless, he considered me to be a dangerous person. Okay.

It was, of course, more than a little bit apparent that VR had not done their homework, either. Anyone who VR has ever sent me to see, about anything at all, has seldom been prepared to talk with me. There's a lot to be said for the prepared listener, I think. For the most part, the people I was coming into contact with back then did not show a great deal of interest in anything I was saying. The year was 1978, and, at the very mention of brain damage, I would find myself bobbing about aimlessly in a sea of red flags. If I were still a drunk, I think I would probably cry in my beer right about now. I knew more about the human brain than most if not all of the VR counselors that have ever been assigned to my case over the years. In most cases, I was only making, at best, educated guesses about my condition myself. But the fact that I was not a dangerous man was just that—a fact, not a guess. (The following statement is a lot more than an educated guess also: The human brain does not have much use for alcohol before or after TBI. Fortunately, and only by the grace of God, I never became an alcoholic. TBI victims: Beware of the grain and the grape!)

The average tax-paying citizen is in the dark when it comes to state programs and their functions for people with TBI. We have what is called "government in the sunshine" in Florida, but I get the idea that the sun only shines when and where the powers that be want it to shine. I'm not trying to be facetious. That is simply my suffered opinion, of course. The Government in the Sunshine laws can be found on the Internet, and you don't have to have brain damage to find them. Of course, only an attorney is able to make heads or tails of them, and I'm quite certain that they're the only ones who ever do.

Here's a fact for you: It's only been within the last ten years that the Department of Vocational Rehabilitation in Florida has even started training counselors to deal specifically with TBI. Remember, I was injured way back in 1963. Rehabilitation programs for folks suffering with brain damage, at least for the average bear in 1963, were all but nonexistent. Rehabilitation for the average bear has slowly gotten better over the years. For the most part, though, access to top-grade rehabilitation remains as invisible as "drain bamage" itself. To tell you the absolute truth, simply thinking about trying to get help on my own makes me feel sick. What a fight—I mean for the average bear, not the James Bradys of this world. Not that I would take anything away from Mr. Brady, whose nickname just happens to be "the Bear." I wish him all the best in his battle with TBI. I know that a lot of good has come to the average TBI survivor because of the Bear's adversity. I only wish this progress could have come sooner and without Mr. Brady's misfortune. Myself, I'm simply the average guy with TBI. And every twenty-one seconds in this country, another average guy sustains a TBI.

I would really love to be given an audience, just one time in my life, made up of all the right people. It would be awfully difficult for me to stop testifying about all of the minds that have been wasted while trying to get help from the State of Florida. Believe me, the right people simply don't want to hear it.

Here's to all the people in this world who have suffered TBI and have had to be subjected to bureaucrats and service providers with far less smarts than they themselves have. The old adage "I have forgotten more than you will ever know," in all too many cases, is a very fitting statement when coming from a person suffering TBI. With one huge exception, of course: In some cases, the person suffering TBI has definitely *not* forgotten everything he or she knows. Not at all. Much of the time, even in the case of amnesia, memory deficits subside over time. In my own case, for instance, I simply have some extremely sporadic and odd assimilation and presentation problems such as neurological confusion, stuttering and stammering and, of course, my on again, off again memory.

The job skills evaluation in 1977 was an absolute waste of time, of course. I remember really understanding, for the first time, what the word "plastic" meant when applied to people. Plastic people! The only thing I was getting from VR was help with my rent, nothing more—nothing aimed at helping me with either my immediate employment problems or my neurological problems. It seemed to me that the only result of my case having been sent to Easter Seals in the first place was in the form of a bill for services rendered. Of course, that bill was sent to VR from Easter Seals, and was paid by the State of Florida.

Evidently there was another consequence. It gave VR one more label to hang on me. (Believe me, they really liked doing that back then, and I suspect now as well. Before VR finished with me, or I with them, more labels were hung on me than bright shiny bulbs on a Christmas tree.) The new label was "low frustration tolerance." That's a really hard one for someone with TBI to disagree with. I did disagree, however, and I was quickly accused of being argumentative and of having some extreme behavioral problems. It's the old "rock and a hard place" scenario. I did ask many people at VR to be more specific. I even requested something in writing pertaining to my behavioral problems, but I never got it. I was told that low frustration tolerance was very specific. I thought to myself at the time, "If that's all these brilliant people can come up with, I'm in big trouble." They had to be kidding if they really thought that by labeling me with low frustration tolerance they were in some way helping me with what they were calling extreme behavioral problems.

Talk about adversity! Believe me, when you have had your bell rung really well there is no escaping it—it's everywhere. Once again, those four P words that I like to throw around every so often (patient, prayerful, persistent perseverance) came into play, big time. From the time I left BBI in 1975 until this very day, my applied philosophy has worked wonders for me.

Of course, I cringe every time I hear someone refer to my faith as a philosophy. Faith and philosophy are as different, one from the other, as the words "objective" and "subjective" are. That bit of information is something that people of all faiths need to remember.

Many professional people over the years have tried to convince me that my faith is nothing more than a philosophy. Be that as it may, I have personally experienced a huge difference between the two. I have certainly tried to understand and show respect for the opinions of others at all times. Nevertheless, a good many of the opinions I have encountered along the way have been absolute garbage. Absolutely! Welcome garbage, but garbage nonetheless.

I didn't receive any help with my affliction or my employment problems from VR until 1989. I was forty-eight years old and the father of two by that time. Finally, VR agreed to help me go back to school. I will tell you this: The fact that I earned an AA degree and my bachelor's degree with financial help from DVR is the only good that ever came out of an otherwise long and arduous relationship. I will say it again: better late than never.

I have heard recently that other states do a much better job with programs for people with TBI and other disabilities. I'm really not sure, and I'm not about to move in order to find out, either. I love Florida. However, in my opinion the Sunshine State is a bad place to be when it comes to living life with TBI.

I have had to learn, often the hard way, to put down my axe and accept the fact that I'm the one suffering with TBI and all the adversity that goes along with it. Some intimidating and insidious laws in the State of Florida hold me in check, so I cannot say anything about the Division of Vocational Rehabilitation of the State of Florida after 1999. In the spirit of putting my axe away, I will say God bless anyone who has ever worked for the State of Florida, and God bless the State of Florida.

The system? What system? No one ever told me that there was a law against my attempts to overcome this seemingly endless Chinese fire drill that I found myself living in. Of course there isn't. On the other hand, there have been many times when I could not find a law that would lend support to my attempts at recovery, either. On occasion I have found the right law. Unfortunately, for the most part it is impossible for TBI survivors to achieve the enforcement of any of these laws. Fortunately for me, the words "surrender" and "quit" did not, and hopefully will not, ever inhabit my vocabulary. Many times throughout my attempted recovery, folks have made the mistake of taking me for some sort of poster boy for Big Government. Nothing could be further from the truth. Believe me, the fish that I have had to fry over the years have had more of an immediate importance to me than my personal politics. I'm really neither a liberal nor a conservative. I count myself as one extremely proud disabled American. (I count, myself!) I am awfully proud of my right to be either a Republican or a Democrat. I take a purely eclectic approach to our form of government. In my opinion, it's the best approach. I like the word independent. It's a fine word. Please call me independent anytime you like.

Exploitation is the word that flashes through my mind whenever I hear about a private program providing help for people who have TBI. In my opinion, and in light of my experiences, they have never done much good, outside of attempting to educate many professional people who should already know about TBI, and more than likely do if their feet are held to the fire. I just don't get it. I have rarely gotten the assistance I needed from a private program. Perhaps I'm totally ignorant of all the good they do for people like me. That must be the case. I hope I am completely wrong, but the private programs I know anything at all about seem to be self-serving. For me to find out that I am totally wrong would be terrific. Please make my day!

The truth is that all social service entities—state, federal, and private—are extremely difficult to deal with. At least in my case they have been, regardless of who was occupying the White House at any given time. The idea of Big Brother watching may not be such a bad idea, especially when it comes to the accountability of programs for the disabled. This is an age of constant change and multiplying choices. That can be for the best, but at its worst, it makes the shifting currents within the social service system hard to keep up with. It would also appear to me that the multiplication of choices in our society has presented "the System" with more to argue and disagree about. Good thing or bad thing?

The things that I have had to learn in order to become knowledgeable enough even to attempt to apply for benefits in many cases, let alone be successful in my attempts, have been unbelievable. It took me almost fourteen years post injury to begin drawing Social Security, and that was only after I had graduated from a school of higher education. Divine intervention played the key role, but I had to learn how to become my own advocate, for sure.

First I had to learn what advocate meant. Then I found I was much better off knowing how to spell advocate, and of course many other words, as well. A study of etymology and semantics has also been really helpful. It all sounds kind of ridiculous, doesn't it? Fighting fire with fire seemed to be the only thing to do. In my case, substituting education and faith for fire proved to be just the ticket. Even with a good education, pinning Social Security down was not at all easy. Every time an application was sent, a form letter came back after what seemed to be forever, informing me of their findings. The findings were always the same, however: insufficient medical evidence. Finally I had to get help from a senator and a congressman before I ever received my first disability check. It seems to me that Social Security never did get my onset date correct. They just might owe me some money. (If they do, they will probably want to pay me back with interest, compounded at that. Fat chance!)

So don't give up. You can always attack in another direction—really! I'm told that applying for help from a state, federal, or private agency is a lot easier today than it was back then. Maybe it is. I certainly hope so.

If I have derived any benefits from state or federal programs other than Social Security, those benefits have always missed my "personal target of need", a phrase I got from a letter I received from one of the state agencies. The disability compensation I have received, both VA and SSI, has been somewhat helpful over the years, and I give thanks to God and to Caesar for it. I have a 30% disability rating from the VA due to the knee injury I incurred while serving a four-year enlistment in the Marine Corps. I have a 100% rating from the Social Security Administration due to my head injury. But my personal target of need, whatever that is, has never been correctly interpreted by anyone. I have never wanted financial assistance nearly as much as I have wanted assistance with my recovery so that I could become self-sufficient. I have had the opportunity to meet many people with disabilities in my lifetime, and most if not all of them would like to be making their own way in life with a job or some type of training that could possibly allow them to maximize their potential instead of feeling as though they were being forced to accept far less. Unfortunately, the powers that be in all too many cases would rather give a disabled person just enough income to barely keep a dream alive, all at the expense of the tax-paying public. I'm not trying to tell anyone that I have never met a person with a disability who has not overcome the odds and become a success, but the fact is that I have met far more who have not than who have. The implementation of the Americans with Disabilities Act is simply not what it should be in many of our great states.

I have always looked for a way to maximize my own potential, even before I had the ability to express that goal. I think we should all do that, regardless of our personal circumstances. A disability should not hinder you from maximizing your potential. Getting out of the ever-so-limiting box that my necessary acceptance of Social Security has put me in has always been my goal. I have made many attempts over the years to improve my life as well as the lives of my immediate family. Most of my attempts to become gainfully employed have improved our lives to some degree. However, a few did not. One step forward, two steps back, as the saying goes. The attempts that did work have always come at precisely the right time, yet seem to have been extremely short-lived. But even my failed attempts have seemingly strengthened our family ties.

Anyway, the opportunities for me to maximize my potential, or at least to move in that general direction, have come solely through my faith in God and not through my faith in any state, private, or federal programs. I'm still working toward maximizing my own potential every day, day in and day out. No Lord, no faith. No faith, no story. Never give up on a good dream.

John Bunyan's book, *Pilgrim's Progress,* was completed in 1684, but it was extraordinarily inspirational in my life. It deals with the paths that the author and his wife chose to lead themselves to heaven. These paths are very trying at times. I can honestly identify in so many ways with his stories, his faith and his thinking. I feel sure that the illumination of my story can be found in the muck and the mire of *Pilgrim's Progress.*

Deeper and deeper I have been stuck in Mr. Bunyan's muck and mire, time and time again. The Lord has rescued me countless times. And now that I have the words needed to express myself, I think I'll give the system my best attempt yet. I firmly believe my faith has only gotten stronger over the years. I know it has. No doubt. Although I cherish help from other people, it is only with God's help that I will recognize and continue to steer clear of any muck and mire headed my way.

The system pertaining to people with disabilities both on a state and federal level is something that is actually there. Really! Just how you might benefit from it, though, is anyone's guess.

My advice is to steer clear of the system whenever possible, but if you do find yourself caught up in it, take what it gives you, but never give up the fight for what you really want or need. My ideas and beliefs along these lines have all come from the many experiences I have had over the past forty years. All too many times along the way, the system appeared to be my only salvation. I'm sure that many of the problems I have encountered within the system no longer exist, however, I believe that the back-biters are still out there today.

The system is there to be worked by you, and you should never stop trying. Never. Most of the state and federal people that I have had to deal with would stop doing anything the minute I stopped demanding they do something. Why? I'm not at all sure. I will tell you this for sure, however: Don't forget to be a squeaky wheel. Remember this also: They seldom call a client. You must call them, and call them often. Take names and kick what?

Another thing that I have learned when trying to get help from these agencies is that they never have enough money. Well, since time is money, I gave them as much of mine as I possibly could. You should try to do the same. It works! It may not work exactly the way you want it to, but what have you got to lose? The human mind is definitely a terrible thing to waste. (Funny how that statement always sounds like such a wonderful one to make even when it's being made by someone who has absolutely no idea what he or she is talking about.)

Over the years I have sent twenty-seven letters to various congressmen and senators regarding the problems I was having with the system, and have received twenty-seven very polite responses from them. I sent the first of my letters in 1975, the year I graduated from BBI. The last letter I sent to anyone citing any trouble I was having with the system was sent in September of 1989, before I found a way to complete my education.

If you'd care to look at those responses, I'd be more than happy to provide you with copies. Unfortunately, copies of letters sent by me over the years have all been lost or misplaced. But the letters of response, by themselves, provide a good deal of insight into my ongoing battle with the system. Certain catch phrases appear over and over again:

"I appreciate your affording me the opportunity to…"
"I want to help in any way I can…"
"I am looking into this matter…"
"I am awaiting a response from…"
"As soon as I hear from…"
"I will be in touch with you…"

Most of the time, the follow up letters were very frustrating:
"I regret that I could not…"
"I know you will find it disappointing…"
"I am sorry that…"
"You may exercise your right to appeal…"
"If you have any questions…"
"If I can be of further assistance…"

But once in a while, I would hit pay dirt!
"I am pleased to be able to give you this good news."
"Your disability claim has been allowed."
"It was a pleasure being able to assist you."

I'm sincerely interested in getting the point across to you that, for a TBI survivor, the only way to get ahead in life is to never give up. That's the same thing everyone else is told when it comes to getting ahead in life. Frustrating, but true. We are all people, damaged brains or not. Everyone is subject to frustration and to the good day/bad day thing to some extent. Faith and education have taught me to never give up.

So never give up!

CHAPTER 10

Where to Now, Saint Peter?

In spite of the system, my life continued to move forward—perhaps not as quickly or efficiently as I would have liked, but forward nonetheless. The education I received while studying at BBI was incredibly important to me—just what I needed to move me down the road toward recovery. I was constantly being challenged mentally. I was forced into competition with others and with myself. I was trying, with all of my being, to use parts of my brain that I had never used before. Best of all, I was learning how to share my burden with God. I was ready to get on with my life, for sure. Where was I going? How far could I go with only my life savings of five hundred dollars, a formal education, an unflappable faith in Christ, and brain damage?

When I first came to Tallahassee, Florida after leaving Graceville and BBI, I remained persistent and hopeful of finding a church to pastor. Of course, finding a wife would be nice, as well. What I was finding out wasn't surprising to me at all. Brain damage is simply not very conducive to finding either one. I had convinced myself that I was in need of more education. Education had almost become some kind of addiction, not to mention the fact that I wanted to be where the girls were. Single females, and the time for anything other than my studies, had been hard to find at BBI.

I decided to go to Florida State University and look up the veteran's contact person. The Veteran's Affairs people were easy to deal with after I told them about my head injury and Baptist Bible Institute. The man assigned to my case seemed genuinely impressed by how far I had already come in my quest to overcome the effects of brain damage through faith and education. He even seemed to be fairly well read when it came to knowing something about brain damage, which is more than I can say about most folks, then or now. Evidently he understood at least something about the misunderstandings and other communication problems I was faced with on a daily basis. He said he could get my VA benefits reinstated if I were willing to work toward a bachelor's degree. Willing! Was I ever!

My timing was right on in September1975 as far as enrollment at Florida State University was concerned. The fall semester was forthcoming. I showed them copies of my transcripts and other necessary papers, and in a few days I was back in school once again.

My education from BBI was paying off big time. That, along with my faith, was enabling me to maintain at least a vague semblance of focus and sanity that was, to some degree, acceptable to the outside world. That old fish bowl of mine was still with me, but my self-esteem was such that successfully venturing outside of it had become routine. (Make no mistake: My old fish bowl is still with me today. What would I do without it?)

Still, I was attempting to study at Florida State University under some very different and difficult circumstances. I recall that after I had attended classes at FSU for about a month, a young woman came straight at me in the hallway following a class, shouting obscenities and going on about Jesus Christ having been a bastard. I was staggered and confused by this unprovoked attack. I offered no response and stood very still. Three or four male students had gathered around and finally I heard one of them say, "Okay, that's enough." I simply walked away. After having spent four years of my life at BBI, FSU bore a striking resemblance to Sodom and Gomorrah. Talk about being a fish out of water—was I ever! (Yes, in my case that was a pun.) It sure seemed to me at that time in my life that being a Christian was much easier at BBI.

Later on, I thought about going to the VA contact person and to the professor teaching the class to report the incident. I was sure the boys had put the girl up to it. At that time, confrontation of any kind was something I absolutely did not need, as, both mentally and physically, I was in pretty bad shape. Maybe I should have said something to someone about the incident, but I never did. What did I say earlier about BBI and their lack of understanding about TBI? Well, FSU was behind the times in their understanding, as well.

One French professor that I had at FSU likened me to a blinking traffic light: now you see it, now you don't. The man simply didn't know just how accurate his statement was. I did. Of course, I was constantly attempting to repair my damaged circuitry. I also knew how much progress I had already made. My light was going to come on and stay on. No doubt in my mind. That blinking light is a lot brighter today than it was back then, and I do a much better job of compensating for the blinking.

The inevitable was fast approaching nonetheless. I had to drop out. The GI Bill had paid my way while I was studying in Graceville, but now at Florida State my attempt at furthering my education came to a screeching halt. Within six weeks of my first class, I was flat broke!

It would take every bit of three weeks before I began receiving a check from the VA once more. This time my timing was not as good. I didn't even have gas money. The Salvation Army and my landlord gave me some help. The last name of my landlord just happened to be Love. That's right, Mr. Love gave me some help and I will never forget it. And the Salvation Army is the one organization that always seemed to be there for me whenever I needed them. I will never forget them, either.

Vocational Rehabilitation would pay my rent at that time as long as I was doing whatever they asked of me, or was volunteering somewhere with the prospect of a full-time paying position at a later date. That's why I was back at VR looking for help. That and the fact that my usage of the four P's seemed to be slipping away a little bit more all of the time, and I simply could not find any work in the Southern Baptist Convention.

Why in the world, after having graduated from BBI, did I need help from anyone? Good question. Exactly why it never occurred to me to go back to BBI for help will always be an unanswered question in my mind. I know I was trying to make all of the decisions necessary for daily living (and all other decisions, as well), through my faith in God. Neurological confusion was running wild and the stress was unbelievable.

That confusion was extremely hard for me to deal with. The neurological, psychological, and just plain physical problems were so intense and so tangled that I actually felt as though my head was about to explode. (I'm sure my head did explode on more than one occasion. Anyway, it sure felt that way.) I remember reminding myself on a daily basis that God was not the author of confusion. It was only my faith and trust in God that gave me the strength to hold things together.

Approximately one week after leaving FSU, I volunteered to work as a chaplain at the Leon County Detention Center for Youthful Offenders. I never received a paycheck, but I always had breakfast and lunch, and my life was going on, for sure. Although I never really felt like the detention center was part of God's plan for my life, I did feel as though I had not turned my back on my calling altogether. After all, I was finally ministering to someone in some capacity. And we shouldn't overlook the certificate of appreciation signed by none other than Governor Reubin Askew, either. (Actually, I have been given more than one such award over the years. Things like that always made me feel good, at least.)

The car I had at that time was not mine. A member of a church in South Georgia was making the payments on it for me until, hopefully, the time came for me to take them over. That day never came. A couple of weeks after leaving Florida State, the man in Georgia took his car back. (Ouch! Things like that *never* made me feel good.) I had been "wheel-less" before, but walking was not at all easy for me. If you ever lose the ability to walk, you might soon learn to appreciate any ability you regain, regardless of how awkward the gait. All I can tell you is that I did what I had to do and, with the Lord's help, whatever I had to do was done.

Vocational Rehabilitation was sending me a check covering the cost of my rent, and I had finally received my first Social Security check in 1976 as well. I left my volunteer job at the Detention Center only after it became clear to me that I was on a dead-end road. My checks from VR stopped. My Social Security checks paid my rent, but left me with little money to buy food or pay other bills.

I remember once when I was paying my utility bill at city hall in Tallahassee, the cashier made the remark, "You have one of the lowest utility bills I have ever seen." I smiled and replied, "I stay in the dark a lot, and I never turn on the AC or the heat." The cashier smiled back at me with an added look of disbelief on her face. Only I knew how true my statement had been. That first year I spent in Tallahassee was a cold one for sure, but it did not compare to the freezing weather I had known as a young boy in Northern Illinois.

I'm certain I began writing this story in my dimly lit and very cold apartment back then. I never did get very far with it at that time. Some unforeseen and totally unexpected events were rapidly heading my way on the last day of 1976, and they caused me to put my story on hold for close to a quarter of a century. All for the best.

I was without a job, without a car, and I had little income. I was still in need of a wife. Many single victims of TBI understand that the need for a spouse becomes exaggerated after their brain injury. I absolutely did not have any idea what was going to happen next in my life. I'm not even going to attempt to explain what was going on with me spiritually at that time. Depression was knocking at my door once more. The only thing at that point that I was absolutely certain of was my faith and trust in Jesus Christ.

It would be seventeen years later, at the age of fifty-one, that I would receive my bachelor's degree. Better late than never! In 1991 I graduated with an associate in arts degree from Tallahassee Community College. In 1992, I earned a bachelor of science degree with a double major in religion and philosophy from Florida A&M (Florida's Agricultural and Mechanical University, FAMU), also in Tallahassee.

Seventeen years is a long time to wait to reach a goal. But once upon a time, some well-informed adult told me that it was all right for me to talk to myself, just so I didn't answer myself. Well, back there in my small apartment I sure did a bunch of talking, not to myself, but to my Lord, and you can rest assured I never once answered my own questions. But all of my questions *were* answered. As for my four P's, patient, prayerful, persistent, perseverance… well, they came screaming back into my life to stay. Those unforeseen, unexpected events heading my way on the last day of 1976 were soon to become some of the most wonderful and outstanding events of my entire life.

Once again, God's grace would put me on the proper path to achieve all of my future goals. When I think back to the day I left BBI, I'm still amazed at how far I have come on five hundred dollars, faith, education, and brain damage.

CHAPTER 11

Holy Matrimony and All Else

Mrs. Brown's lovely daughter is what happened next. Twenty-three years old, Mary Nell Brown was a very nice, yet unexpected and totally unpredictable occurrence. I'm not saying I didn't believe my prayers would be answered. I was simply blown away by the how and the when of the whole thing. Sometimes I really do question God's timing. I shouldn't and I know that. Mrs. Brown's lovely daughter was the worst thing that could have happened. She was the best thing that could have happened.

There I was, trying to find a church to pastor, and at the same time I was becoming extremely convinced that God might have other plans for my life. What might those plans be? I didn't know. The things I wanted to take place in my life had not been happening fast enough, or at all. At least that's how I saw it. Any patience I had left was certainly not mine alone.

What to do? I wanted to do something productive with my life, so I decided to tell my story. I began to write about my life. I felt sure I was doing the right thing. Just putting it all on paper and knowing that there wasn't anyone to stop me was awfully exhilarating. At the time, you might say that writing was more like some strange type of dictation for me. I heard this voice in my head—Walter Cronkite? Roger Mudd? I'm not sure, but whoever that commentator-like voice belonged to, it was extremely helpful. I believed then, and believe to this day that that voice and its rhythmic ramblings had been sent from on high to aid me in my writing.

Then, on New Year's Eve 1976, my apartment doorbell sang out. (That's USMC talk for rang.) Startled by the unexpected sound, I dropped my pen and quickly turned off the voice in my head. That voice was a true blessing, but the ringing of my doorbell would soon prove to be a blessing on a much larger scale.

"It's open!" I called out, and with that statement reverberating around my small, dark apartment, the door flew open and in stepped someone who would become one of the three ushers at my future wedding. (What wedding? Hang on! We'll get there.)

"Let's go celebrate on the top floor of the round Holiday Inn tonight." I was slightly taken aback by his request. After all, this guy was a member of the First Baptist Church of Tallahassee, and had been for most of his life. He was also a senior at Florida State and was about to finish up there with a bachelor's degree in humanities. I looked at him intently and inquisitively for a moment. "You know I can't do that," I replied. "Yeah! And I shouldn't either," he said, as he shrugged his shoulders. "But were going to go anyway"

Well, like the man said! Anyway, in about one hour's time there I was, once again, sitting on a bar stool, reluctantly sipping on a shot of "Jack Daniels" on the rocks—a very refreshing taste. I was in some extremely familiar surroundings indeed. The reluctance I felt toward the whole situation seemed to be mitigated in some peculiar way, and not just by the obviously intoxicating effect of the Jack.

I really was reluctant. I truly wanted to leave before I ever even got there. What was I doing? At the same time I had my ever-present feeling of peace, and the insistence of my small inner voice that everything was going to be just fine. (If you have never heard voices, maybe you should. Or perhaps you should simply own up to them. Look out now! They're coming to take us away!)

Suddenly I realized my good friend was gone. He had been sitting next to me, and above the never-ending noise, we had gotten fairly deeply into a humanitarian and theological conversation. We had been having an ontological discourse from a humanitarian point of view. Then the guy vanished. He more than likely simply had to go. (Beer, you know.)

Sitting there alone, I could just barely make out three people coming my way through the smoke, noise, and revelries. Party, party! One young-looking man, in the company of two equally young women, was obviously looking for a place to sit and place their drink orders. Both of the young ladies were fairly attractive—early twenties, I thought. One of the ladies (the smaller of the two) was obviously the girlfriend of the male in the threesome.

I assisted the guy in his attempt to order drinks. They all remained standing. My friend never came back. The idea of not having any way to get home never dawned on me at the time. Strange, but I never gave it a thought. I introduced myself to my new friends, and they did likewise.

I felt as though I was having my usual communication problems, and the Jack Daniels was beginning to have a numbing effect as well. The immediate effects of alcohol on a TBI survivor are extraordinarily exaggerated in most cases—and that's very true in mine.

The obvious couple moved off toward the dance floor. I asked the young lady, they had left behind, if she would like to dance. The noise was so intense my slurred words went undetected. I also felt confident that I would receive a negative reply to my request. I had overheard her tell the other girl she did not feel like dancing. I really didn't want to attempt standing at that point. I had more than one reason, of course.

She moved toward the empty stool. The next thing I knew, this creature was sitting on the bar stool next to me—the one that had become vacant with the disappearance of my good friend. This chance meeting, if you want to believe it was that, became something more the very first time our eyes met. She had these big, blue, intriguing eyes—striking, I thought. She had a wholesome look as opposed to the racy look that I was accustomed to seeing in bars. As we talked, the fact that both she and I were slurring our words above the noise was actually comforting to me.

We both knew it was almost time for the ball to drop in the Big Apple. Together we found the dance floor. Dancing was not easy for me. My spastic moves seemed to fit in just fine, however. I had learned from experience to fake it. Faking it always went well when it came to dancing. By concentrating on the rhythm I could take the extra steps I need to take in order to keep from falling.

We both seemed to enjoy each other's company. I was both satisfied and pleased with the things I was able to find out, in conversation, about this person. I was actually beginning to hope she had similar thoughts. She was obviously of good character. Her values seemed to be in line with mine, and when I talked about Christ, her countenance seemed to become visibly brighter. She struck me as being both knowledgeable and bright. She had an obvious sense of responsibility about her, and I particularly admired the fact that she appeared to be a mature and sensible being. I also sensed a certain vulnerability that I felt was somewhat alluring, but at the same time I believed this vulnerability to be well within her control. She told me she had become a Christian at a young age but still had many questions about religion.

I can't say this was a case of love at first sight. I can't even say I thought she was my type—I really didn't care much for the way her hair was fixed. But by that time I had gone through so many changes due to TBI that I really was uncertain as to what my type of *anything* actually was. I realized, however, that my interest in this woman was definitely peaking as the last few seconds of '76 rapidly slipped away. The ball finally dropped and we kissed our first kiss. The friends who had been with her when I first saw her offered to give me a ride home. Of course I took them up on that! I was not at all sure what was happening, but my newfound friends, all three, had expressed a genuine interest in getting me home safely. They did.

I asked them in. I wanted to give them some of what I considered to be the very best, most mouth-watering London broil I had ever prepared. We all ate until the steak was no more. They all said it was good. (I sure wish I could remember how I did that. Shoot! I wish I could always remember how to do whatever it was I did yesterday. I bet I haven't done anything the exact same way in years. TBI can lead to innovation and innovation can lead to a variety of successful ways of doing things.)

We all talked in an attempt to become a little more acquainted. I left out the part about my faulty memories, innovation, and all of my successful ways of doing things, in hopes of having the chance to tell the young lady in my company all about it at a later date. In the wee hours of the first day of the New Year the sandman finally crashed the party.

It was after noon when I awoke and began moving about. Actually, it was already after 3:00. You may rest assured that on the first day of 1977 this old boy had a new set of questions stomping around in his damaged gray matter! Would I ever see those people again? One of them had left me with a strange feeling of unfulfilled interest. Curiously, though, I was content in believing that somehow my interest in that blue-eyed charmer was mutual.

Wait! Darn it! I didn't even get a phone number. Thoughts of the kisses and the closeness of our short time together persisted. Who was she? I prayed. Lord, if this is your will, please let me know more.

There was a phone in my apartment when I moved in, and the manager of the complex had helped me get a working number since I didn't have the necessary deposit. But, like I said earlier, I hadn't gotten anyone's phone number the night before. Maybe, just maybe, someone got mine. I was sitting on a kitchen stool, next to the phone. Back to the drawing board, I told myself. (My kitchen cabinet was doubling as my desk, i.e. my drawing board.) I was lost in deep concentration. The welcome voice in my head had once more established a rhythm, and my pen was trying to keep up with my every word. After all, writing (becoming a starving writer with absolute hope as my subject matter) was what I had decided to do with my life before that interruption on New Year's Eve, 1976.

The intense concentration of that moment was short-lived. The phone sang out. (USMC talk again!) In an apparent reflex action my hand shot toward the phone. Wait, I told myself. Let it ring a couple of times at least. I picked it up. "Hello," I said, "who's calling?" The answer came slowly. "It's me, Mary Nell."

TBI rapidly look over, and for an instant confusion reigned. "Mary who?" I stammered. "This is Mary Nell Brown. You know, from last night." I told myself to speak slowly, and try to sound very deliberate. My ministerial tone might be helpful. "Yes. Mary Brown. I remember. Of course I do."

"Mary Nell, Joe, Mary Nell is my name."

"Mary Nell Brown. Right! I had trouble with that all last night, didn't I?" I said in an apologetic sort of way. "Yes, you did," she said with a nice little giggle—not silly, just sweet. Her voice had something more than the usual Southern accent, something different—extra-sweet sincerity. Down-home sincerity? I think I was in love with Mary Nell's voice right off. She said the sweetest things in the sweetest ways I had ever heard.

"I lost one of my earrings last night. Will you see if you can find it for me, please?"

I thought to myself, the age-old earring and sofa ploy. But this lovely person quite simply didn't have a clue about that. "Yes I will, I'll look right now. If it's here I'll find it, I promise." And I eagerly added, "I'm going to call you right back; I know you gave your phone number to me last night, but I…but I…well…"

Before I completed my flimsy explanation my pen was moving once more, only this time I was trying to keep up with a lovely voice—the sweetest sound I ever heard in my life. Thank you, Lord! I got her Number!

I found the lost earring. I called her back. Shortly after that we became inseparable. We talked many times about what we wanted our future lives to be like, and what our beliefs and values were. I had already been living with the results of traumatic brain injury for fourteen years or so at the time of our marriage. I had indeed come a long, long way in my attempt to recover from TBI by 1977. I told my wife-to-be all about the accident in 1963, and we discussed it many times. I did my best to explain the effects of brain damage, but any in-depth understanding of TBI by either one of us was something that would have to be left in God's hands. We were both falling in love.

I guess love really is blind and a little on the hard of hearing side, as well. At that point and time in our lives, neither one of us was giving a lot of rational thought to the adversity we were sure to face in the years to come. (I remember reading someplace that at least 90% of all decisions made in this world are made in accordance with emotion rather than rational thought. Think about that.)

Mary Nell Brown had graduated from Leon High School in 1971. She went to work for the State of Florida as a Clerk Typist I within two months of completing high school. She has moved up the pay scale very nicely over the years. She is now forty-nine years young.

My wife is a very intelligent person. She has always had her head on straight and her feet firmly planted on terra firma. Without my wife's dedication and loyalty to our family, none of us would be where we are today. She has stayed the course through some very rough seas. "TBI riptide" is what I like to call it. What I am really talking about, of course, are all of the adverse situations spun off from, or created by, the fact that I have had TBI throughout our relationship.

I have been led to believe by some neuroscientists that when under prolonged stress, a person's brain actually shrinks. If what those scientists have said is correct, the results of a totally objective study of my brain would find not only damage, but a severely shrunken brain to boot! (My experience has more than taught me that the answers to all of life's extremely demanding questions are to be found in a totally subjective study.)

Feel free to call me crazy. In all honesty, I've stopped counting the number of times someone has called me crazy. Besides my mom's references to cows, she was always saying, "They told Christopher Columbus he was crazy, too." I'm not really sure who "they" were, but I got her point. (Please don't try to tell me the word crazy didn't skip across the retina of your mind's eye when I was telling you about the voices in my head. I mean, after all, how sane can a guy with TBI be? It's your call!)

When my sanity is questioned, I love to tell folks this: I have found myself staring four different types of cancer straight in the eye, along with the residuals of TBI. Please don't try to tell my wife and me that we have not learned to live through an ongoing nervous breakdown. Stress, stress and more stress! I should be dead! If not for the Lord and my wife in my life, I would be dead—very dead! Insanity! I wonder where I'd be today if I had settled for mere insanity.

I in no way expected my wife to be mysteriously capable of helping me deal with my problems in any other way than I was already doing, and had been doing for years. She actually did, though. She still does in so many different ways. Come to think of it, my wife and her ways were and are a bit on the mysterious side, at that: companionship, intimacy, and something called love! Once again, patient, prayerful, persistent perseverance is what it is all about. (I love being able to tell you about this stuff... what a connection!) There are not enough words in the English language to tell my wife how much she has meant to me over the course of our marriage. I will always be extremely thankful for having her in my life.

For the last twenty-six years, my wife has been caught up, to a large extent, in the same storm I seem to have been riding all of my life: adversity, adversity, adversity. The only true calm or peace in that storm has been found in knowing God. He has always been there for us, and I am certain he will be there for us for all eternity.

It wasn't fate that brought us together. It was faith. Faith is what keeps our marriage from total destruction. I have done some crazy things over the course of the last twenty-six years. The road traveled has not been without some extraordinarily deep potholes, and peaks and valleys nonstop. Things like forgetting to put the cap back on the toothpaste can't compare to what I've done, or forgotten to do. Come to think of it, remembering to do the small things has never been much of a problem for me. It's the big things, like remembering to control my anger and knowing what my life is all about that have been the challenges. Remembering the names of other people has been a chore, and that alone has not been at all conducive to the cultivation of friendships. I have on occasion forgotten my own name, phone number, and address. On the same occasions I have been able to recall with uncanny accuracy many other things both learned and experienced. I have not forgotten things as much as I have seemingly misplaced them in my consciousness. Do you understand what I'm saying? What has been most problematic for me is just how sporadic my recall can be. My wife doesn't try to figure it all out, and she doesn't nag me about anything, either. My wife is great. She works overtime to accept me as I am.

Just as my wife knew about my brain damage, she knew about my faith in God, as well. There was no doubt, as far as I was concerned, that he would be with us every step of the way throughout our lives. I believed then, and I believe now, that our marriage on the ninth day of July, 1977 was definitely part of the Lord's plan for both of our lives. I realized from the beginning of our relationship that without an abundance of faith in God and in each other, our relationship would be the worst thing that could possibly happen to either one of us. I can't count the number of times divine intervention has saved our marriage. We have always argued like Democrats and Republicans, on occasion even worse. It has always taken collaboration for us to find consensus in our conflicts, and of course the Love of God has always been with us.

Our marriage met with very little approval from the get go. At the beginning of our relationship, I was not liked very much at all by the in-laws. But over the years many people who are close to us have seen us face our troubles and overcome them every time. I think I've won them over. Faith, discipline, hard work, and a definite sense of responsibility plus my 4 P's have proven themselves to be hard to argue with. Success is always hard to argue with, as is adversity overcome.

Mary Nell Brown was unexpected, unpredictable, and out of the blue. I hope I can get away with using that worn-out cliché—

it's a perfect description! A chance meeting at best is perhaps the most understandable way to describe the way my wife and I met. I don't see it that way myself. No, I really don't. I see it as the grace of God, and a relationship that, through faith, will last an eternity.

My wife was born in the only hospital in the Capital City at that time: Tallahassee Memorial Hospital, also known as TMH. Both of our children would be born there, as well. Looking back on the day when my wife told me she was pregnant with our first child, although I can't remember everything about that day, I do know my first reaction was one of thanksgiving and extreme joy. Of course, just how I was going to pull this parenting thing off would soon be given over to my faith in my God. I had been given a good deal of instruction along the lines of parenting while enrolled at BBI. However, with my recall inconsistent at best, just as it has been in all other areas of my life, it took a lot of faith for me to find the peace of mind it takes to raise two children today. TBI does not add anything to any relationship. My wife, my kids, my faith! Divine intervention and human instrumentality! I have had more help spiritually with my life since my acceptance of Christ than most people want to hear about. Our family dynamics can be summed up in one word: faith. Make that two words: faith and devotion.

I'm certain that by becoming a family man, husband and father I was truly taking a very big chance. The chance I was taking with marriage in the first place was by no means an odds-on favorite for success. I did not want to hurt any other human being in any way, but I was well aware of the potential I possessed for doing just that. Who really knew what to expect? I knew better than anyone just how far from being the "average Joe" I had come, so any kind of average family life would be very hard to achieve. But nothing ventured, nothing gained! Lead, follow, or … or what?

Our firstborn, our daughter Erin, is twenty-four. She has played organized soccer since she was six years old. At the age of fourteen she began to play soccer for a team that was sanctioned by the FYSA (The Florida Youth Soccer Association). She also earned a four-year letter and many other awards in high school, and was a member of the National Honor Society. Unfortunately, Erin tore both of her anterior cruciate ligaments, the right one twice, before her eighteenth birthday. She went from Tylenol to Demerol overnight, and she still refused to give up the game. She's a tenacious little redhead with a nose for any goal. Given a soccer scholarship, she attended Flagler College in St. Augustine, Florida, and was given an award for being the only woman in the history of the school to play soccer all four years. She earned her bachelor's degree at the age of twenty-two. Any prouder I could not be.

Our son Stephen is twenty-one. He's attending Tallahassee Community College, and hopes to transfer to Florida State University in the not too distant future. Perhaps the single most important thing my son has learned thus far is that one accomplishment is worth all of the intention in the world. (I said it here but I'm sure someone else said it first.) Stephen is a gifted athlete with one large problem: He was born legally blind. At this time his vision cannot be corrected. Stephen is somewhat beyond belief. He insisted on being mainstreamed in the public school system. (Sibling rivalry has been extremely intense in this household!) I like to tell myself that my son has learned to see not by sight alone, but by faith. I can tell you this much for sure: His father will never stop praying to that end. He earned a high school letter as the back-up place kicker for his school football team, of all things! It's awfully hard to imagine, given the adversity my boy is faced with, that he could ever wind up kicking a football in college or perhaps even for a living one day, but we all know stranger things have happened, don't we? Never give up on a good dream!

Our family dynamics have always been extremely success-oriented. Of course that fact has always been in large part due to my own quest to be normal—the average Joe once again. Hopefully the above-average Joe! I have always relied on my faith in God to keep me from going overboard. My success in that area? It depends on whom you ask and when. Challenges and problems have absolutely become the norm in our household, many of which are well-documented problems and challenges that occur in most other families as well. It's like I said earlier: Most everything seems to become exaggerated when you suffer brain damage. The really unique challenge for all of us has been learning to understand and forgive the guy with TBI.

I recall a day, a few years back, when someone brought a magazine article into a psychology class that I had been taking at the community college in our city. He read it aloud, and as I recall (I'm sure you have gotten the drift pertaining to my recall by now) the person who had written the piece was obviously steeped in child psychology. The article really impressed me. After another 30 minutes of discussion on the subject, the class ended. I hurried home, trying hard to hold onto my take on what I considered to be some impressive information. I immediately called both of the kids into the dining room and we all sat at the table. Erin was about twelve years old and Stephen about nine. I positioned myself at the head of the table, of course, and said, "I want you two to understand something and it's something very important. I want you both to know that I'm doing the best I can do when it comes to raising you. However, I may not be doing everything just right. You both may turn out to be neurotic messes but it's extremely important to me that you both know I'm doing the best I know how." Just then my wife stepped into the room. My son's request was first and fast: "Mom, can I go back to my room now?" My daughter had a lost-in-thought look on her face as she followed her younger brother's lead. I was left standing there repeating, "Do you understand what I'm saying?" More often than not I have felt it necessary to say whatever I'm thinking before I forget it, especially if I feel that "whatever" is important. And just like most other people, most everything I say seems important at the time. Whatever!

While I have been the overbearing disciplinarian, my wife has been the indulgent one, and although neither one of us may have understood the other's stand completely, somehow we have managed to hold the family together. That ever-so-important balance has come through for us in all matters, and not only in the raising of our offspring. I have found that relationships never seem to work very well in fifty/fifty mode. Fifty/fifty in my state of being is simply not the way to go. Collaboration and win/win certainly worked for us. Both of my children respect me, although each in his or her own way, and I thank God that somehow I have been able to earn rather than demand that respect. My kids even come to me on occasion for advice. How about that for faith?

The way both of my children have been able not only to relate but also to understand me to any acceptable degree is nothing short of miraculous. Through all of the ups and downs we have experienced, love has prevailed. Living with me or anyone else who has suffered a severe head injury is not easy. Just ask my wife. She often tells me that she does not have to read my book—she has lived it. Our children feel somewhat the same way.

Mary Nell and I had been married about ten years when my mother died in 1987 of lung cancer in Georgia. Georgia, of all places (her words)! She said she never liked the name Georgia.

The lung cancer that claimed her life was caused, more than likely, by smoking a pack of Camels a day for sixty-odd years. Smoking a pack of Camels a day for sixty years is more than enough to kill anyone (my words).

My half sister and I, in keeping with the earlier request of our mother, threw her ashes into a swift-moving current of air at the top of Wayah Bald, her favorite spot in North Carolina's Blue Ridge Mountains. She told me once, before she became sick, that if we did that for her and if she were lucky enough, her ashes would be blown all the way to Pike's Peak. "These mountains are just a bunch of hills—beautiful hills, but hills nonetheless." She had a special love for Colorado and the Rocky Mountains.

My mother left some money and some property to my sisters and me when she passed away. Of course, my wife's state income as well as a small business venture have helped us a great deal as well. We as a family have been able to maintain at least a semblance of upward mobility. We have made numerous sacrifices both together and personally over the years in order to create the family and middle-class lifestyle we now enjoy. It is extremely hard for me to imagine anyone getting ahead in life if he or she is unwilling to make sacrifices. Many times, when faced with obstacles, we have found personal sacrifice to be a necessity. Our faith in God has, without exception, been the source of our strength.

Adversity has certainly not been a stranger to my wife or my children. When I think of how they have overcome setbacks thus far in their lives, my belief system is reinforced one hundred times over, and I'm still counting—counting the blessings. My convictions have become stronger, and the word pride does not begin to express what I truly feel, not even a little bit!

EPILOGUE

Here we are at the dawn of a new century, and I find that I have this compelling need to write about my entire life and my understanding of what I believe to be divine revelation in it. I'm sixty-two years old and some things seem to be slowing down. Of course, time itself remains fleeting. I have lived with TBI for forty years.

Now that I have become a senior citizen, the fog which has surrounded me for years seems to have become a bit less dense. That feeling of being on the outside of something looking in is much easier to deal with nowadays. The confusion is gone for the most part, and even when it's not, peace always prevails.

I don't believe that neurologically I have gotten much better over the years. I wish I could tell you otherwise. I do know for sure that I have had to consciously and constantly act in an attempt to adapt to my surroundings, but I've always had to do this. Sometimes it can be just a bit tiring. I could have and would have just as soon sat down...

I don't expect you to know what that really means unless, of course, you happen to be a person who has experienced the same thing in your lifetime. There are still times when I feel like someone is chasing me. However, thanks to God and Satchel Paige, I'm not about to look back now. I thank God for the abundance of personal resources he has given to me over the years. The ability to compensate in so many ways and for so many different things has been so great—unbelievable!

I have been able to maintain a certain super zest for life throughout most of my extraordinary never-ending recovery. I have also been given the faith and strength it takes for a TBI survivor to live a productive life. Life has been the absolute best for me and life has been the absolute worst for me. I have had one far-out ride.

Living life with TBI really has beaten the alternative. Of course, we could become involved in a deep theological discussion over that statement, but please, not today! If I have learned anything in life, and I believe I have, it's simply this: Life is not always fair. The rain falls on the just and the unjust alike. We all face adversity at one time or another. Some of us are faced with more adversity and some with less. Life goes on. How we create an understanding for, and an acceptance of, the complications in our lives is the key to overcoming them.

I simply do not, in any way, believe in luck. For me, luck does not exist. Neither bad luck nor good luck exists. Patient, prayerful, persistent perseverance. The four P's are where it's at for me. In my opinion, overcoming difficulties of all shapes and sizes is directly connected to our knowledge of all things and our faith in God. I am definitely a believer in the idea that in all adversity there can be found opportunity - a silver lining, so to speak. But I know I don't think exactly like everyone else in this world—not at all! That can be and has been well documented.

Today I'm living a very successful, happy, purposeful, significant, and extremely productive life, and I feel very satisfied with it, for sure! Do I still face adversity? You bet I do! There will always be a degree of difficulty involved in everything I do, either mentally or physically. But I no longer face any of the challenges of life alone. Examining the past revelations of my life has led me to believe that dealing successfully with adversity can be, and in many ways should be, an ongoing process. I am exceedingly pleased and ever-so-quick to tell you that forgiveness also seems to have been critical to my success. Learning to forgive others is important, and learning to forgive yourself is imperative.

Through it all, I have remained one very proud, extremely happy-to-be-alive individual. I got to be a husband! I got to be a daddy! I own my own home! We even have two dogs and three cats. I have become well-rounded, well-adjusted, and well past insanity, I hope! I have been and will be misunderstood forever. It comes with the territory. The stuff I have learned while stumbling through life with brain damage has brought me much closer to the true stuff of life. Ambiguous and paradoxical, maybe. But that's life!

I am certain of one thing more: I really would love to do it all again without brain damage. But so what? The American dream has been realized here for sure, and love is always in the air!

APPENDIX A:

TBI Basics

I believe it is of some importance for you, the reader of my little book, to have gained a good understanding about TBI in general when you put this book down. If this story causes you to protect your bell a bit better than I did mine, then I have truly done a service for mankind.

No two cases of traumatic brain injury are exactly alike. What has happened to me as a result of having had my bell severely rung may or may not happen to the next guy. I suppose it would be truly amazing if any of us could find someone who has had exactly the same experiences in life. We are all unique, one from the other, but at the same time we are all very much alike, brain damaged or not.

I recently found a list of what were called possible brain injury deficits. There were twenty-three of these deficits listed. I would like to pass them on to you.

Possible Brain Injury Deficits

- Contracture deformity *+
- Depression **
- Bowel dysfunction
- Bladder dysfunction
- Urinary tract infection
- Cardio-respiratory impairments*
- Personality changes**
- Behavioral changes**
- Activity level changes **

- Memory deficits **
- Sleep pattern changes *
- Problems in interpersonal relationships **
- Social withdrawal **
- Identity problems *
- Headaches *
- Vertigo **
- Irritability *
- Loss of interest *
- Loss of emotional control **
- Learning deficits *
- Language problems *
- Intermittent periods of anger or temper *
- Aggressive acting out *

* I personally experience these symptoms to a mild degree.
** I experience these symptoms to a moderate to severe degree.
+ Deformity of a limb without discernable primary changes of bone. Basically, this means the limb does not work right.

If you have recognized many of these symptoms in yourself or a loved one, I urge you to consult with your doctor as soon as possible. What you may have thought was just another bump on head could, in reality, have been much more. I have experienced all but four of the deficits found on this list myself, and a few more that are not on this list as well.

Many of the deficits that I have experienced have only mildly manifested themselves in my case. You might think that's a good thing. Wrong! When it comes to my brain injury, more often than not the mild manifestation of a deficit has caused me the larger problem. Many times, what makes recovery from TBI so tough is the fact that you simply can't give up and resign yourself to some of your milder neurological deficits. Believe me, all too often you're damned if you do and you're damned if you don't.

Brain damage has often been referred to as the invisible disability or the silent epidemic. You may call it anything you like. I hope and pray you never experience it. But TBI is not always invisible and it's not always silent. TBI is never "always" anything or any particular way.

TBI is the number one killer of young adults in America today. It could happen to you or someone you love in the twinkling of an eye. Today, every twenty-one seconds, what happened to me forty years ago is happening to someone else. And that's just here in the USA.

From what I understand, it is not possible for medical science to repair or rebuild brain cells at this time even though it has recently been discovered that it is possible for the brain to generate new cells. Protective head gear for everyone—that day is on its way. Not at this time, but that day is on its way.

APPENDIX B:

TBI Statistics

The following statistics were all obtained from Centers for Disease Control publications.

- Every 21 Seconds, one person in the U.S. sustains a traumatic brain injury
- In the U.S. in 1995, direct and indirect costs of TBI totaled an estimated $56.3 billion (Thurman 2000).
- Each year in the United States, an estimated
  - 1.5 million people sustain a TBI, which is 8 times the number of people diagnosed with breast cancer and 34 times the number of new cases of HIV/AIDS (see graph below);
  - 50,000 people die from a TBI, which accounts for one-third of all injury deaths;
  - 80,000 to 90,000 people experience the onset of long-term or lifelong disability associated with a TBI.

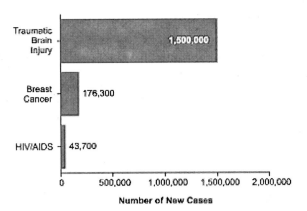

Incidence of Selected Health Problems in the United States

Data Sources: Traumatic Brain Injury 2001 (CDC), Breast Cancer 1999 (American Cancer Society), HIV/AIDS 1998 (CDC)

- Brain injuries are among the most likely types of injury to cause death or permanent disability.
- Among children ages 0 to 14 years, traumatic brain injury results in an estimated 3,000 deaths; 29,000 hospitalizations; 400,000 emergency department visits.
- An estimated 300,000 sports-related brain injuries of mild to moderate severity occur in the United States each year.
- At least 5.3 million Americans, or 2% of the U.S. population, currently live with disabilities resulting from TBI (Thurman 1999). (This estimate is based on the number of people hospitalized with TBI each year and does not include people seen in Emergency Departments who were not admitted to the hospital, those seen in private doctor's offices, and those who do not receive medical care.)

- The leading causes of TBI are vehicle crashes, firearm use, and falls (Thurman 1999).
- Crashes involving motor vehicles, bicycles, pedestrians, and recreational vehicles are the primary causes of TBI (Thurman 2001).
- Firearm use is the leading cause of death related to TBI (CDC 1999).
- Firearms cause about 10% of all TBIs, but they account for 44% of TBI-related deaths (CDC 1999).
- Nine out of 10 people with a firearm-related TBI die (CDC 1999).
- Nearly two-thirds of firearm-related TBIs are classified as suicidal in intent (CDC 1999).
- Males are about twice as likely as females to sustain a TBI (CDC 1997b).
- People ages 15 to 24 years and those over age 75 are the two age groups at highest risk for TBI (Thurman 1999).
- African Americans have the highest death rate from TBI (Thurman 1999).

APPENDIX C

TBI Resources

If you would like more information about traumatic brain injury, please contact:

- The Brain Injury Association of America
  105 North Alfred Street
  Alexandria, VA 22314

  Phone: 1-800-444-6443
  Fax: 703-236-6001
  http://www.biausa.org/

- Neurotrauma Registry
  P.O. Box 440
  Hunt Valley, MS 21030-0040

  Phone: 1-800-373-1166
  E-mail: info@neurotraumaregistry.com
  http://www.neure.com

Traumatic Brain Injuries can occur for a variety of reasons. With that in mind, other sources of information include:

- Centre for Neuro Skills
  2658 Mt. Vernon Ave.
  Bakersfield, CA 93306
  Phone: 1-800-922-4994
  http://www.neuroskills.com/

This is an excellent website with many articles and research updates on brain injury.

- The Tammy Greenspan Head Injury Collection
  http://www.nassaulibrary.org/farmingd/TamaraGreens
  panHeadInjuryCollection.htm
  If you visit this site and e-mail the trained librarian, you may request that a free book on brain injury be loaned to you.

- Lash and Associates Publishing
  www.lapublishing.com
  An excellent site on pediatric brain injury, offering great tip cards, articles and useful information.

- www.Dana.org - the Dana Alliance Group. They have a great deal of information on brain research of many different types. Another great resource they offer is the "Brain Connections" book, a book that lists hundreds of organizations that work on the behalf of different brain disorders, from Alzheimer's to Tourette's Syndrome.

- Bicycle Helmet Safety Institute:
  4611 Seventh Street South
  Arlington, VA 22204-1419

  Phone and fax: 703-486-0100
  Website: www.bhsi.org

- The National Center on Shaken Baby Syndrome
  2955 Harrison Blvd., #102,
  Ogden, UT 84403

Phone: 1-888-273-0071
Website: http://www.dontshake.com/

- National Resource Center for Traumatic Brain Injury:
  http://www.neuro.pmr.vcu.edu/

- Traumatic Brain Injury Survival Guide:
  http://www.tbiguide.com/

APPENDIX D

Lake Bluff Orphanage Reports

D-1: ChildServ Report—Summary of Joe's Records

Lake Bluff Orphanage is now part of an organization called ChildServ. When I requested my old records, they were happy to provide copies. They were also kind enough to summarize the intake report. So for those of you who don't wish to read the more long winded pronouncements from the early 50's, this report should give you a good overview of my stay at LBO. It's also interesting to see how cautious and tactful social workers have become in the past fifty years. Compare this to the original intake reports, and you'll see that back then they didn't pull any punches!

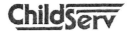

8765 W. Higgins, Suite 450, Chicago, Illinois 60631
www.ChildServ.org
773.693.0300   FAX 773.693.0322

June 9, 2002

Joseph Thomas Blakemore
6713 Pasadena Drive
Tallahasse, Florida, 32317

Dear Mr. Blakemore:

This letter is in response to your request for history of your residence
at The Lake Bluff Orphanage from August 17, 1951-August 15,1953.

History of Placement

Your biological mother was 35 years old and separated from your
father, also 35, at the time of your placement. She was working and
renting a room for herself while paying for your care in private foster
placements. She believed that the fact that you had had to move so
often was creating a problem for you and your sister. She wanted
consistent care for the two of you at a place where she could visit
with you regularly until she could implement her plan for the three of
you to be reunited.

She was concerned that you had had to repeat a grade due to
multiple moves one school year. She worked with agency staff over
a period of time to research the best way to go about exploring the
idea of placement at Lake Bluff Orphanage. With your mother's
permission, you and your sister visited prior to placement. You came
to live at Lake Bluff on August 17, 1951, when you were ten years
old.

Your record indicates that you were able to get past your initial
sadness. Your mother visited regularly, and despite your initial

HELPING CHILDREN BUILD BETTER LIVES SINCE 1894

ACCREDITED

explanations to your little sister that you would be with the boys, you were always available to her and seemed to be a real support for her.

You worked with the adults to participate fully in the school, residence and camp programs. You had athletic ability: You were a baseball player and an archer, as well as a horseback rider while at camp. It seems you didn't much care for water at first but took swimming instructions and made marked improvement.

You were obedient and helpful and had an interest in getting along with adults and children. In the residence you lived with older boys. You were just at that age where you could go with one group or the other. Your mother reported that you'd had older friends with whom you had enjoyed playing so you moved in with that age group. You got to know each other and within a few weeks you seemed to have settled into the routine of things.

Your Health

Your mother reported that you had Measles at age 6, chicken pox at age 6 and mumps at age 9. At age 7 you had a tonsillectomy. You had a blood Wasserman test with negative results on 8/7/51; a scarlet fever vaccine in 1944, a diphtheria test/inoculation in 2/42, and a TB test with negative results on 8/6/51. You took a whooping cough vaccine in 2/42. Your vision test of 1951 was normal. The doctor stated that you had a normal physical on 8/6/51.

While at Lake Bluff Orphanage you had an appendectomy at Lake Forest Hospital on 3-31-52. Your hemoglobin count was low over the next several months and you were prescribed iron treatment and monitoring. Reports indicated that you made progress and were predicted to continue to do well provided you took iron capsules (2/53).

Education / Vocation & Interest

Your mother had had you repeat a grade prior to your contact with Lake Bluff. Her concern arose for your success in school after you had some difficulty with your reading scores during a series of moves that involved changing schools. Your previous records had indicated good progress so she reported that she thought it would help you going forward. It appears that this proved helpful as your final school report the following year showed a normal reading score. You had an overall average in the C range with some grades above and some grades below.

The conversations your mother had with the staff throughout the time she worked with them to plan for your care always focused on how long it would be good for you to live in institutional care. They settled on an estimated two-year timeframe, and that is what eventually occurred. In August of 1953 your mother made arrangements for you to move to the home of your paternal uncle (8/17/53).

....

The above non-identifying information regarding your biological parents was retrieved from your placement records. Please keep in mind that this information was completed by the Lake Bluff Orphanage caseworkers in 1951-1953. While it is ChildServ's desire to provide you with accurate information, we cannot guarantee that it is without error.

I hope that this information is helpful to you. Sally Almen is looking into the brochure you mentioned. She will contact you with the result of her search. Please contact me, Mary Pat Clemmons, at 773-693-0300 regarding any information or clarification you might need.

Sincerely,

Mary Pat Clemmons

J. T. Blakemore

NAME: BLAKEMORE   PAGE: 1

Mrs. Blakemore called on this date, enquiring about institutional placement for her nine year old boy. IW stated that
LB would consider the child for care but would not be able
to begin the study for a couple of weeks. Mrs. Blakemore
said that she was not certain about the child's need for
immediate placement at the present time and planned to talk
with the boy's present foster mother on a private basis who
is ill to see whether or not this foster mother will be able
to keep him temporarily until she thinks through further
placement plans. Mrs. B. was to call IW back. Since she
had not called at the end of the month, IW considered application a withdrawal and closed case on 8-22-50, destroying
record of her notes. During this original contact, Mrs. B.
stated that she had been referred by ICH&A. On 6-25-51,
Mrs. Blakemore called again regarding institutional care for
her boy and girl. She is still living at her former address
in Westmont. Her telephone number remains the same and she
states that the best time to call her is any day before 10:30
a.m. in the morning. This time Mrs. Blakemore stated that she
had been in touch with Rev. Harold Taylor of the Methodist church
in Downers Grove and he had talked to her about LB. Mrs. B.
said that she had been in touch with us about a year ago but
had not called us back since she had found a private placement.
No agency is at present active with her, although at one time
she had been in touch with Family Service in Glen Ellyn and
Miss Deeds had given her some help regarding suggestions for
places to place the children. Mr. Blakemore had deserted about
three years ago and has not been heard from since. Mother is
a waitress and supporting herself and children.

IW accepted the two Blakemore children for study on this date (6-25-51)
and made an appointment to talk with mother at LBO on 7-2-51.

Mother came to LB according to her appointment. She began by
saying that her children had moved around a great deal and up
until the present she has been "fairly fortunate in finding
good foster homes." Both children need to be moved from their
present foster home situations at the present and Mother feels
that they no longer should be having a series of foster home
placements but should begin to call one place home. She feels
that she should have begun to think of institutional placement
about five years ago, instead of this late.

Mother came out strongly against court placement and said that
other agencies she had contacted, such as ICH&AS, had told her
they only handle court cases and so they would not have anything
to do with her since she refused to go through court. In 1950,
during the month of August, Mother had had an interview at ICH&A.
She felt it was perfectly all right for IW to clear with ICH&A
regarding this. ICH&A at that time referred her to LB and to the
Protestant Children's Haven. After Mother had worked out a private
placement for her children, she got a letter from Protestant

D-2: LBO Intake Form—Joe and D-3: LBO Intake Form—Judy

These two reports, which were compiled at the time by the social workers, doctors and administrators of LBO, reveal a great deal about the time my sister and I spent in the orphanage. I have added a few footnotes for the sake of clarification.

NAME: BLAKEMORE   PAGE: 2

Children's Haven, stating they were able to consider her application. Mother stated that she had been discussing LB and the
Protestant Children's Haven with several people since that time
and prefers to have the children here at LB.

At one time, Mother telephoned the welfare office at Du Page
county in Wheaton, Illinois, and they had suggested various
schools where she might place the children. At present, the
boy, Joey, is with his uncle on his father's side. Mother
began to cry when she talked about the conditions in the home.
She felt that this brother and his wife had recently developed
some trouble between them and were not getting along too well.
She also said her son needed to sleep in the attic and she
felt pretty badly about that. She explained how she was very
touchy about anything concerning children and was quite concerned about the many moves the children had had to make and
their inability to feel completely at home in some of the foster
homes they have been in.

Mother is working at Bill's Restaurant at Cass & Ogden Avenue
in Westmont, Illinois. She has been there over three years and
works from 11:30 a.m. 'til 8:30 or 9:00 at night, sometimes later.
The telephone number of this restaurant is Downers Grove 1087.
She has been paying $10.00 weekly for each child for the past
five years. Her husband does not support at all. He hasn't been
heard from for the last three years. Even his relatives don't
know where he is. Mother felt that he wasn't a lazy person but
did a great deal of work but apparently just didn't assume the
responsibility of a home and supporting the children was not too
much of a concern to him now. She feels that if the relatives
did know where he was, they would tell her. She feels that there
might be some possibility, even, he would be sick or have ailment
in which he couldn't be making an adequate enough living to send
money for the support of the children. Mother makes about $50.00
weekly and gets all her meals there. She rents a sleeping room,
but would like to have an apartment where she could have the children with her occasionally. She isn't able to take the children
in her sleeping room.

In talking about some of her problems in placement, she brought out
how one of the foster mothers had liked her boy so well that she
had wanted to adopt him. She felt that it was almost inevitable
if it was a good foster home they would want to adopt the child
and then the child would have a tremendous conflict of loyalty
between his mother and his foster mother.

Financial arrangements in lieu of a placement at LB were discussed
somewhat. Mother felt that she had been doing a good job of supporting the children all this time and felt that she could continue to
do this. She did not feel she could rely too heavily on relatives
and did not have any other resources. She has no savings or insurance. IW brought up the question of what if she should become ill
or something else should make it impossible for her to support the
children. She seemed to take the view that getting ill just hadn't

219

NAME: BLAKEMORE   PAGE: 3

happened to her very much so she didn't too much count on it
happening now.

IW did not press financial arrangements further at this time
because Mother seemed pretty set on her ability to support the
children without any outside help.

Mother told about being referred to LBO by Rev. Taylor. She
knows Rev. Taylor through her work at the restaurant and also
because her children have gone to his church some. Mother did
join the Methodist church as a child but doesn't attend now
because of the work. She was somewhat apologetic about this.

Mother definitely has Illinois residence but IW did not go into
establishing this since IW was aware during this interview that
she would not be continuing with this intake study.

Mother felt that she had a good relationship with her inlaws
but that they were not a source of support for her.

Mother brought up her problem of discussing the possibility of
placement at LB with her children. She didn't use the word
"Orphanage" in discussing it with her children and later she
heard her boy say, "I hope it isn't an orphanage!"

An appointment was made to continue the discussion regarding
placement plans at LB on July 9th at the Chicago Temple.
                                                    CE:ev

During interview on this date, IW received some school records
from mother. Permission was granted to keep these records for
a time during the intake study but they are to be returned to
mother later.
                                                    CE:ev

Review

Second interview with mother. IW met mother at the Chicago
-Temple on this date. Mother was dressed very attractively in
a spring dress with a straw hat and straw purse to match. As
usual, she makes a very good appearance. She was considerably
more poised during this interview than the previous one. She
had been a little "weepy" during the last interview but she
seemed quite controlled and calm during this interview.

IW saw a birth verification on Judy. This verification was a
letter dated 2-24-44 from the county clerk of Lake county,
J.B. Morse, saying that they had a record of the birth of Judy
Lynn Blakemore at Condell Memorial Hospital, Libertyville, Illinois,
on 10-22-43.

Judy will soon be going into the third grade. She has been doing
better than B average work in school. She did have kindergarten
experience prior to beginning first grade. She is attending the
Downers Grove Public School, called the Longfellow School. Mr.
Jack Elzay is the Superintendent and her teacher is Mrs. Diener.

1. They quote me as saying, "I hope it isn't an
orphanage!" When I figured out that it was I was
devastated. I just couldn't comprehend it. But my
disappointment and displeasure was tempered with the
realization that before this, I didn't get to go to the
YMCA every week, and would never have had the
opportunity to do things like go horseback riding. This
was all great fun for a child my age, so I learned to
accept it.

NAME: BLAKEMORE   PAGE: 4

IW saw a Bureau of Census Certificate from Washington, D.C.,
stating that Joseph T. Blakemore, the son of G. Barnes and
D. A. Blakemore, was born 7-1-41. Mother states that "T"
stands for Thomas. Joseph is known as "Joey" by the family.
The Bureau of Census Certificate number was 12357, and the
certificate states that Joseph was born in Pikes Peak, Colorado.
Mother stated that she was in Pikes Peak at that time because
she was following her husband around the country. He was one
of these persons who continued to travel about after their
marriage. Mother stated that some men drank and some men
traveled and she wondered which was worse. She indicated that
the reasons for her leaving her husband were largely tied up
with his constant need to travel around and inability to settle
down and establish a home. IW did not go into this further
and actually discouraged her talking about it at this time
since IW will be stepping out as the intake worker very soon,
another worker taking over.

Joey will be in the fourth grade next year. He is one year
behind his regular grade. During his second grade he made a
great many moves and so at the close of his second year in
school mother had him put back into the first grade and then
the following year he repeated the second grade again. His
reading is still quite poor, although his other subjects are
average.

Again IW discussed a possible court placement with Mother and
after considerable discussion, Mother agreed to a court placement and was actually able to see certain benefits in this.
It was agreed by IW that when our study was almost completed,
our intake worker, Mr. Whitaker, would get in touch with the
Du Page county Juvenile Court and assist Mother in making a
referral and final hearing through this county. IW feels it
would be helpful if Mr. Whitaker took some responsibility in
interpreting the need for a court placment to the Juvenile
Court in Du Page county in order to make it easier for Mother
to go through this experience.

IW discussed the change in workers from Miss Enzinger to Mr.
Whitaker and Mother seemed to accept this with considerable
ease. It was left with Mother that Mr. Whitaker would get
in touch with Mother as soon as he was able to continue the
intake study. Mother mentioned that the relatives with whom
Joey was staying were going on a vacation the last part of
July and although it was not absolutely necessary to have plans
worked out for Joey at this time, Mother felt it was highly
desirable if they could be since she hated to have Joey make
another move. Throughout IW's two interviews with Mrs. B.,
IW found her very cooperative to work with and very sensitive,
discerning and warm in her efforts to make more adequate plans
for her children.

According to arrangements worked out with Mother, IW
visited the two Blakemore children at LB on this date.
They were brought to LB by Rev. Devore and Mother's
landlady. Mother's landlady felt that the children
might be strange coming alone and since their mother
needed to work on this day and was unable to come with
them she decided it would be a good idea for her to come.
Rev. Devore has known Mrs. Blakemore casually and was
willing to make the trip for her.

Since both Blakemore children requested that IW take
them on a walk to the lake, on this date, IW walked
down and back with the two children, discussing topics
with them.which they brought up, not initiating many
new subjects. Both children related quite quickly to
the worker,not in a warm, attached manner but in a
friendly, casual,conversational way. They seemed
interested in learning about L.B. but did not appear
frightened or unprepared for this visit. They understand
that their mother is thinking in terms of a placement at
LB for them. Joey appears to be quite an active, out-going
little boy with interests similar to other boys of his age.
He enters actively into group activities in his neighborhood
and talks enthusiastically about the various sports activities
of his play group. He is small and slightly built for his age
but states that he plays with boys older than he is most of
the time and prefers this group. He seems sensitive about
his size and possibly tries quite hard to over-compensate
for his small stature. In talking about his activities, it
appeared as though he was quite a capable, alert child in
his play. He appears pretty strongly attached to his *play group*
in his present neighborhood and wonders whether or not the
boys at LB will like him. He showed quite a disinterest in
girls and a strong affiliation with boys and boys' activities.

Joey talked quite freely about enjoying school but mentioned
that some subjects were kind of hard for him. He seemed very
sensitive about being a year behind other boys his age and
explained it by saying he had moved around so much once that
he needed to repeat a grade. In talking about his difficulty
in learning to read, he brought out that there were other
subjects he could do pretty well and almost as well as the
rest of the boys in his class. *IW felt "Joey" showed
considerable aggression in his general behavior.*
Judy is a well-dressed, well-groomed, poised, very well-mannered
lady-like kind of girl. She is quite sensitive to good grooming,
clean living quarters and cleanliness habits. She talked very
politely to the worker but showed considerable freedom in expressing her feelings irregardless of the negative nature of
these at times. She appears to be much more free in expressing
herself verbally than Joey. She takes somewhat of a maternal interest in
Joey, correcting him at times and being a little alarmed by his

2. I have no recollection of my mother not being there
    when we were dropped off at the orphanage. I have no
    explanation for this other than the fact that she was
    very pragmatic person. She constantly adjusted her
    priorities to produce the outcome that was best for
    everyone. In her mind, to take off work was to lose
    tips, and she couldn't have that. And she had come
    with us when we first visited the place, so this wasn't
    our first exposure to LBO. We had been through so
    much with our father, and had been moved from pillar
    to post so many times, that this didn't seem like a
    major, life changing event to any of us.

NAME: BLAKEMORE   PAGE: 6

poor manners and general boyish behavior. Judy appears to
be quite self-sufficient, but having a capacity to relate
pretty warmly to adults and children her own age. She also
was interested in hearing more about L.B. and expressed an
interest in coming here. Joey seemed a little more reticent
about the plan.

IW did not go into a description of L.B. unless in specific
answer to the questions of the children.   She explained
the reason for her seeing the children at this time but assured them that the decision as to their coming was still indef-
inite and whatever would be worked out regarding permanent plans
would be done so with the mother and she, in turn, would discuss
the permanent plans with them. IW pointed out both she, the IW,
and/mother were interested in Joey's and Judy's reaction to L.B. and wanted
them to help participate in making the decision. The children
appeared to understand why their mother is unable to have them
with her at the present time although IW wonders if they still
do not feel that a plan of living with the mother might be a
possible one. They are pretty accustomed to being separated
from her, however, and having her work and visit them on her
day off. She has explained to them that she cannot care for
them and support them by working at the same time and so it
has been necessary for her to place them.

IW talked briefly with Rev. Devore on this same date and
learned that he had considerable feeling against the placement
of the Blakemore children because he felt there were other
children in the neighborhood who were more closely affiliated
with the Methodist Church than the Blakemore children were.
He thought that L.B. should give preference to those children
although he admitted that these children, namely the Joyce
children, were not ready for placement at the time. He thought
he would have difficulty explaining to his parishioners why
the Blakemore children were taken instead of the Joyce children,
although, he at least intellectually understands why L.B. is
doing this. Rev. Devore had considerable feeling about L.B.
taking non-Methodist children into their center.   CE:ev

According to an interview arranged by Mother, IW met Mother
at the Chicago temple on this date. Mother discussed the
children's reaction to LB as being a favorable one, although
she felt the children certainly have some reticence about
going to a new place. In discussing the possibility of placing
Joey in the older boys' hall, Mother felt that this would
definitely be preferable since he prefers to play with older
boys and tries very hard to keep up with boys in the grade
ahead of him or boys his own age even though his size is
smaller. She feels that he gets along very well with his
play group and Judy with hers.

Mother is a high school graduate, having finished in the
home town in which she grew up. Her husband had two years
of high school. The children have always spoken English

J. T. Blakemore

in the Blakemore home.

IW discussed at length the referral to the Du Page County
Juvenile Court on this date and discussed ways in which
mother might proceed with a referral through this court.
Mother has been quite reticent all along to accept this,
but now seems willing to go ahead. She wonders what sort
of experience she will have in court and is somewhat
dreading it, but feels that at least one of the Probation
Officers knows something about her situation and will be
sympathetic to her case. A conference including IW, Miss
Enzinger; case workers, Mr. Gale and Miss Simmons; new IW,
Mr. Whitaker; Group Work Supervisor, Mr. Maier; Superintendent,
Miss Brooks, was held on this date. Miss Powers and Mrs.
Whitaker were seen separately by Miss Enzinger. The Blakemore
social history was reviewed with IW giving reasons for placement and reasons for considering an institutional setting for
the children. There was general agreement in this conference
that the Blakemore children should be accepted for placement.
                                                          CE:ev

IW talked with Mrs. Duncan, P.O. of the Du Page County
Juvenile Court, telephone, Wheaton 8-2300 on this date. She advised
that Mrs. Blakemore should come to her office and she, in
turn, will introduce Mrs. Blakemore to the State's Attorney,
who will file dependency papers. The hearing can be arranged
as convenient. IW made arrangements to attend this hearing.
Monday or Thursday afternoons are days when hearings are
scheduled. Mrs. Duncan explained that the guardianship of
children placed by Du Page county remained in the hands of
the P.O. and the agency received custody.   CE:ev

Mother brought the two children to L.B. on this date.
IW talked very briefly with the children and then spent
considerable time with mother. Consents for Child to Ride
Bicycles and Wesley Memorial Hospital blanks were signed on
this date. These are filed in their usual place in the record.

Mother feels that Joey would really prefer to live with her.
He seems to have a stronger need for this than Judy, at least
at the present. Occasionally her children urge her to marry
so that they will have a Daddy and she will be able to stay at
home and not have to work to support them. Mother has spent
considerable time discussing with them the reasons why they
have needed to be placed all these years and the reasons why
the present placement plan is being considered. Mother feels
that in two or more years she may be in a better financial
condition to maintain an apartment and support the children
with her income since the children will not need/close supervision at that time. Her own mother will probably be drawing

NAME: BLAKEMORE   PAGE: 8

Social Security Old Age and Survivors' Insurance by this time
and would not need to depend upon mother for support as she
would need to do if mother took her own mother with her to
live now. The paternal grandmother is 67 years old but is
quite active/in her age. Mother feels that Joey might suffer from
lack of male companionship but he might be able to get in with
men with whom he can identify in the neighborhood in which they
live. Mother feels that the maternal grandmother gets along
with boys pretty well and doesn't make a girl out of them.
She, however, does not seem to get along with her husband and
does not live with him.

IW mentioned briefly that mother should probably consider that
the children might be more of a supervisory responsibility in
a few years than they are now. This might be particularly true
in Joey's case. It is also possible that mother's financial
situation would not be able to improve in the ensuing years.
Mother feels these are possible developments. She apparently
is not planning too far into the future, at the present time,
and may have some rather unrealistic thinking involved in her
future plans, though her present plans for the children seem
fairly well-grounded in reality.

Mother discussed Joey's reading difficulty. She feels this is his only
main difficulty is school. The teacher has petted Joey considerably. The teacher even admitted that she did this. Mother feels
that the children have been favored all the way along in school
and have not been given enough chance to face reality. She feels
that the school has sort of handled Joey as a problem child and
have been afraid of upsetting him. They rather handled him with
kid gloves. Mother said that once Joey came home and said something about having been kicked around and she answered back to
him firmly: he really hadn't been kicked around, but he had been
in good foster homes and the people, in general, had been very
considerate and understanding of him. Mother feels that he him
should be allowed to capitalize on what he has heard about being
kicked around and not having a father, to be with him now. Mother
feels that one of the values she would like to have in institutional
setting/give to her children in a more realistic concept of life.

Mother is very agreeable to Joey's receiving tutoring if the tutor
has a good relationship with her son. Mother made her contacts
with Downers Grove School in order to get more information regarding
the children's school adjustment. IW learned that Joey has had
no kindergarten experience. His first grade was spent at the
Westmont School. He showed normal progress in this school.
According to reports mother received from the school superintendent
and secretary there, Joey had taken a reading test toward the end of
his first year and received a normal score. He spent his second
year from September until January in the Downers Grove School
and then spent about three weeks in Dexter, Iowa. From there
he spent a part of the second year, through March, in Des Moines,
Iowa. At the end of March, he moved back to Westmont and it was

225

NAME: BLAKEMORE   PAGE: 9

at this time that Mother put him back in the first grade
feeling that he had had a very poor second year. She knew
that she was moving him around in more schools this year
and regretted it, but felt she was unable to do anything
else because of the family problems. Joey repeated his
second grade again at Westmont and spent his third year,
his past year, in Westmont School, too. He did normal
work in those second and third grades. Mother feels that
he likes it all right but takes a more active interest in
sports and social activities with the boys.

Mother feels that her children should not be pushed in school
but she is satisfied if they do normal work. She thinks B
and possibly a C are sufficiently good grades for the children.
She mentioned that she went through school at the head of her
class but she didn't exactly feel that that was too advantageous.
Mother appears to be more interested in the social development
of her children than the academic.

Mother feels that Judy is much more sensitive to getting better
marks than is Joey. She tries hard to get better than the other
children in her class. Judy has had a year of kindergarten
experience. This was one-half day school. She spent her first
grade in the Westmont school and was given a reading readiness
test toward the end of the year. She passed this very well.
She spent her second grade at Downers Grove, and will be
going into third this fall. She has done above average work
in school. Up to this time she has had women teachers who have
been very fond of her, and tended to pet her just as the
teachers have done with Joey.

Mother came out very definitely in saying that Judy's cute
and everybody knows it. She showed a great deal of pride
in talking about her daughter. She felt that Judy should be
given a more realistic picture of how to get along with people,
however, and to be helped so that she does not use her looks
so much in attempting to get things from adults. Mother feels
that Judy has certain resentments against being petted by
adults but IW wonders if actually Judy doesn't really enjoy
this sort of attention from adults. Mother feels that people
have always thought Judy was very attractive and have given her
too much attention regarding this. IW discussed how the children
might find it difficult to share with other children in the institution and to particularly share the attention of adults.
Mother feels that since the children have been spoiled by foster
parents at times and that Judy is pretty good at being able to work
adults and has been allowed to do so, these are definitely not
realistic patterns and they need to be broken down somewhat.
IW feels that Mother is not punitive, at least not too obviously,
in her attitude concerning the value of an institutional placement
for her children but actually is quite able to see desirable values
in such a placement, and understand how a group setting can

3. At first glance it may seem harsh that my mother describes us as "spoiled" and as "not having a realistic view of life." After all, the two of us had been bouncing from one home to another. But my mother bent over backwards to make sure we had the material things. If we wanted a new toy, doll, baseball, whatever, she'd get it for us. Therefore she considered us spoiled. Because we had material things, she didn't think we were deprived. In her view, having no father or home was terrible, yes, but it wasn't going to deprive us of having a positive outcome in life.

contribute to the growth of the children. IW feels somewhat
that Mother may sense her own inability to help the children
face life more realistically and is actually, on an unconscious
level probably, wanting support from stronger adults in handling
this situation with her own children. IW feels that the children
have probably demanded too much of this mother and she really feels
that she, too, is guilty of "spoiling" them and being unable to say
no to their demands even though a no would be more valuable to all
in the long run.

Mother makes roughly from $210.00 to $220.00 a month as a rule.
She gets most of her meals at the restaurant where she works.
She rents her room in a private home at $25.00 monthly and oc-
casionally eats breakfast there. She does not pay additional
for her breakfast but furnishes the lady with whom she lives
with certain breakfast supplies occasionally. She is not able
to have the children for an over-night visit at this home but
the children are familiar with mother's landlady.

Mother has three separate insurance policies on herself. One
of these is a straight life policy. She carries one policy on
each of the children and one on her father. This one on her
father was begun some years ago and the insurance company
has advised her to continue it rather than drop it. The total
insurance premiums amount to $10.00 monthly. IW suggested that
she might want to review her insurance plan with Mr. Gale, case
worker, some time. Mother stated that Prudential is coming out
with a family medical plan and she is interested in this. IW
stressed strongly the value of a medical insurance policy.

Mother has a telephone in her room but does not have metropolitan
service. This costs her about five dollars monthly.

Mother spent considerable time in working out her own clothing
budget and a clothing budget for the children. She wears uniforms
to work and rather expensive play shoes for work. These shoes,
she feels, are most comfortable. She wears a pair out about
every three months and these shoes cost her about $10.50 apiece.
She feels that shoes are one of her most expensive items but she
feels this item is very important since she is on her feet so much.
She doesn't sew her own clothing but does sew some of her children's
clothing. She believes a low estimate of her clothing is $12.00
monthly. It was difficult for her to give an estimate on her
children's clothing, but she thinks it is about $20 to $25 for both
children, including only three seasons in the year: fall, winter
and summer. Joey wears a narrow heel in the shoe size. He has a
very flexible arch and has difficulty getting a fit for his feet.
IW and mother discussed the value of Mother supplying the children's
clothing or having LB furnish it. Mother feels she would prefer
LB furnishing the clothing and she'll pay a monthly allowance for
this. She feels she would like to buy extras for the children,
however. Whenever these extras occur the CW can feel free to
discuss this with the mother. Mother brought out that Joey is
not particular about the clothing he wears. Judy is quite fussy
about her clothing. Mother will discuss with the children this
clothing arrangement made with IW.

J. T. Blakemore

NAME: BLAKEMORE   PAGE: 11

Mother walks occasionally to work when the weather is nice
but does need to take a cab at times. She is not near bus
transportation so uses a cab quite frequently in getting to
town and back or in visiting the children. In estimating
the cost of weekly round trips from Downers Grove to L.B.,
and her own transportation to and from work, mother believes
she will need about $20.00 monthly for transportation.

Since mother does not eat at the restaurant for most break-
fasts and eats out during her day off, she estimates this
expenditure at about $15.00 monthly for food. Miscellaneous
allowance of $10.00 a month is allowed in mother's budget.
Mother takes a vitamin supplement which has been recommended by
her doctor. This costs $4.00 monthly. She has lots of diffi-
culty with arthritis in the spine and has recently spent money
in treatment of this. This did not give any relief so she
thinks she will not bother with treatment of it any more. Her
general health other than that is good.

Mother spends about $3.00 monthly for laundry. Her medical and
dental is estimated at $5.00 monthly. A $6.00 monthly allowance
for recreation and money to be spent on the children was put in
mother's budget. It was recognized that this was a very small
amount to cover this expense.

IW discussed court placement through Du Page county with mother
and made plans for mother to go to Du Page county to file for
a dependency hearing. It was agreed that mother would pay $40.00
monthly child care rate on each child, and in addition, a $15.00
monthly clothing allowance for both children. This would bring
mother's total list of expenditures to $105.00. This gives her
a slight allowance in case she runs over on some of her items,
but it also leaves some possibility for mother to save a little
money. Mother feels that that would be extremely desirable, if
possible. She has no savings at present, but is accustomed to
keeping a small amount of savings.

Mother has been paying $10.00 weekly for each child for their
basic care and in addition supplying clothing for the children.
She feels this arrangement with L.B. should be able to allow her
to save a slight amount each month. It was agreed that mother
would review the budget with the case worker whenever she felt
this was indicated, and at the same time the case worker could
feel free to discuss this budget with her if case worker felt
it might be possible for mother to pay more toward the support
of her children.

On the basis of the above budgetary computations, it was agreed
with mother on this date that she would pay to the Du Page county
court $95.00 per month for both children. This $95.00, $47.50 per
child, is to be the total child care rate. It is understood that the
$80.00 is the minimum rate required by the Du Page county and the

228

NAME: BLAKEMORE   PAGE: 12

$15.00 extra was figured as the possible addition that
mother could pay toward the support of her children according to the present budgetary figures. The case worker,
however, can feel free to discuss extras or unusual expenses
with mother and of course the $95.00 child care rate for both
children does not include unusual medical expenses. It does
include the regular medical services that apply to L.B. children.
Regular clothing, allowances, scout dues, etc., are considered a
part of the services given under the child care rate and other such
expenses which are due to all LBO children through the child care
rate.

On the basis of this interview, and previous interviews with mother,
as well as with those attending the Intake Conference and those
with other LBO staff involved in the intake decision, IW accepted
the children for placement on this date. Mother will discuss this
decision with the children and also plans for continuing placement.
Further intake plans for the children were discussed. Mother has
her one month vacation beginning this week so she will be free
to cooperate as fully as possible with LB placement plans. She is
considering a change in jobs at this time, also.
                                                CE:ev

IW met Mother and Joey at the Chicago Temple on this date.
As usual, Mother is always prompt to appear for her interviews
and carries through on plans discussed in previous interviews.

Mother appeared in court to file for a dependency hearing on
8-6-51. She stated that she had told Mrs. Duncan that L.B.
agency was not ready for a hearing but they went ahead and had
a hearing anyway and "placed" the children at L.B. as of August
15th. The P.O. had told mother that if placements were not
possible by this date, it would be easy to change them.

Mother is considering changing jobs; she would like to be closer to
L.B. and may be able to make more money in another waitress position,
at the same time bring herself closer to the children so that it will
be more convenient to visit once weekly. She wondered whether
or not this would affect her residence in Du Page county and IW
stated that this should be cleared before placement of the children
occurred. IW will take the initiative in doing this. Mother seems
fairly satisfied in doing waitress work in a reputable place,
primarily, however, because it is most remunerative for her. She
feels she gets along well with customers and is quite a good
waitress. As she expresses it,"If there's a tip, I can get it."

4. "If there's a tip, I can get it." I love this quote, because
it shows what a formidable woman my mother was! In
other parts of the report, you'll notice that she was also
very insistent about paying our fees as well as my
hospital bills and summer camp. She felt it was
important for her to adhere to the material things. In
our chaotic lives, she could control the material, at
least.

J. T. Blakemore

NAME: BLAKEMORE   PAGE: 13

IW left it with mother during the intake discussion
that mother would visit the children once weekly on
her day off, at present, on Monday, unless some other
visiting arrangements are felt advisable. If so, CW
could feel free to discuss this possibility with mother.

Mother does not pay income tax at the present time. With
the support of the two children and her estimate of her
yearly income, it has not been necessary for her to make
these payments.

Mother's parents are at present separated. However, they

did not effect this separation until their children were
grown. They never did get along very well, but did not do
too much fighting between themselves. It was more a matter
of vastly different interests and ambitions. Mother grew up
in a small rural area. She lived for a short while on a
farm in her younger years and then spent the rest of her early
years in the small farmer town. She went to grade school and
high school in this small town. Her father managed to lose
three farms. He was a good employee when working for someone
else but did not have the ability to go into business on his own.
For a good number of years in his latter employment years, he
worked for the John Deere Hardware Company in this small town.
For awhile he suffered with Bright's Disease at that time and
since that time he has done farm-hand work. Later, he developed
an arthritic condition. Now mother feels he is probably on Old
Age Assistance or possibly he is receiving some Old Age and
Survivor's Insurance. He lives with his own mother in this small
town. The Blakemore children see him about once a year. The
maternal grandparents see each other occasionally on family
get-togethers. They are quite formal to each other but do not
object to being at the same gathering at the same time. Mother
feels they are better off separated. She feels that her father
is a very good-natured, easy-going, intelligent person.

Mother feels that her own mother has a personality a lot more like
mother's. She was a school teacher prior to marriage. She was
much more ambitious than her husband. Like mother, she is geared
to a pretty fast pace, is ambitious, energetic, and has her time
occupied with a good many activities. When mother was younger,
she took her own mother's part, but now that she is older, she
realizes that her mother nagged her father a good deal of the time
and that her mother is partially responsible for their inability
to get along. At present, the maternal grandmother works in a
cafeteria on the salad station in Des Moines, Iowa. Mother pointed
out an incident when the maternal grandmother was 62 and she went
and got a job in a restaurant although she had never worked in a
restaurant before. Mother felt that her own mother had a reputation
for stretching a dollar further than anyone in their small town.

230

NAME: BLAKEMORE   PAGE: 14

The family was very poor but tried hard to give their
children a good deal. Mother would like to give her own children
more than she was able to have when she was younger, but she does
not feel that material things are too necessary for children's
development. The children see their maternal grandmother about
once a year. Mother still feels that the MG and the children
could have a fairly good relationship with their grandmother
when living with the mother and/helping to care for the children.

Mother thinks differently now about the importance of men to her.
She does not think she will be likely to remarry although IW
feels this might not be really what mother desires to happen.
She talked, however, about how the children press her for
marriage so that they will have a home. She felt that she
would like to remarry if the person she married would make a
good father, but as a rule, she doesn't feel the men she dates
would really be able to accept children from another marriage
and this would not be a valuable relationship for the children.

Again IW and mother reviewed the long-time plan for the children.
Mother thought that placement at L.B. was indicated/at least two
years. She hopes the children will get a   better picture of
the way things really are. "They have been in homes where people
have taught them quite a bit but they need to learn more about
getting along." Mother feels sure she has over-compensated for
their lack of being with her by buying more than she could actuall
afford. She feels that inter-play in a group situation will be
very good for them.

Following mother's high school graduation, she worked about two
years, in the small town in which she grew up, as a telephone
operator. She had a very good work record with this company.
Then she and a group of girls went to Des Moines to seek their
fortune, so to speak. She began working in a restaurant at
this time and has been in the restaurant work most of the time
since then. However, she did not work during parts of her
married life. She met her husband while working in a restaurant
in Des Moines.

Mother knew that her husband had been married once prior to
their marriage. She stated she believed the court had ordered
a small support for the child from this first marriage of her
husband. This support order was probably about $2.50 weekly, and
it was kept up by Mr. Blakemore for some time. However, when he
heard that his first wife had re-married, he stopped paying the
court order although he did not consult any court about this
action. The mother worked in waitress work or in department
store work until the children were born. During this time they
moved all over the country. Her husband would work a short
while in a place and then move. Mother talks about this
tendency of her husband to move about the country as his chief

negative as far as a/husband and father. She felt that
some men drink and some men move around. A chef does
either one or the other. They were married almost five
years before the children came and got along fairly well
during this time. Mother feels that if they had not had
children and if her/husband not had the added responsibility
of being a father, they/could have gotten along very well
Mother, however, wanted to have a family and to settle
down and have a home of her own. This her husband never
agreed with, on a real emotional basis, although there were times
when he would grant this request to mother, but not carry
through. He supported the family well and was very good
to the children, but he seemed to react to them more as an
older brother rather than as a father. He was quite immature in his ways and lacked the strong personality of his
wife. He seemed to love his home but could not stay in one
place. He was more likely to maintain casual contacts with
neighbors rather than develop intimate relationships.

After Judy was born, the difficulty became more intense between
the parents. Mother thought that some of their problems could
be solved by/a home and at this time, since her husband was
working in Chicago, they bought a home in Round Lake. At first
her husband would get home on week-ends and sometimes during the
week but then he came home less and less, eventually. There
were other relationships maintained by her husband during this
time but/Mother strongly feels this was not one of the primary
reasons for their beginning to grow apart. He more or less
took on these other relationships because he could not meet
the demands of his family. Mother feels that Joey, particularly,
grew close to her husband and that Judy knew him slightly.
Judy took a more negative attitude toward her father, however,
and would often resent his being around or hold off her father
from getting too close to her. This hurt her father quite a
bit.

Father has not seen Joey or Judy since prior to the parents'
divorce. Joey was about five and Judy about three when they
last saw their father. It appeared harder for Joey to have
given up his father than for Judy because he knew his father
and got along well with him. He has some need to idealize
his relationship to his father. Mother felt that Joey sensed
something wrong in their relationship, even though he was a
small child. She said that she and her husband did not quarrel
in front of the children, however. Prior to the divorce, the
Blakemores were separated for awhile and father would send
about $50.00 weekly. After the divorce went through in January,
he sent $35.00 weekly until spring and discontinued support pretty
much from there on. He did not worry very much about the children's
welfare because he felt that his wife could do most anything and
could take care of the financial needs of the children because she
was so very capable.

In January, the year following, the divorce, mother went/down to

Florida with the idea of working for awhile to get some
money. She made her first private foster home placement
at this time, leaving them first with the wife of a former
employer of hers whom she had known in Chicago and later
working out some placements for the children with friends.
She accidentally learned of her husband's whereabouts in
Florida and went to talk to him about getting some support
for the children. He agreed to give some at this time and
finally/into re-marrying him, stating that the situation
would be much different this time and that he would settle
down and make a home for the children. However, they lived
together only a few weeks and mother realized that her husband
had not changed any and would not provide a home for the
children. They separated and mother came back to Chicago.

The children have had about five foster home placements
during their life time. One of these placements was about
a year and a half and it was the only placement in which the two
children were together. Mother felt that this one particular
home still has very strong ties to the children and mother
wonders about the advisability of the children continuing to
see these people. She feels the children actually are in
conflict about where their parental loyalties lie. They were
very much more so when they were in the home. These foster
parents wanted a great deal to work out adoption plans. IW
suggested that mother discuss this with case worker, when
possible. Mother is quite distressed about the children
having had so many placements and this is one reason she is
particularly eager for an agency placement.

On this date, Joey got quite impatient during IW's long
interview with mother and part of the interview was carried
on in a soda fountain, part of it in the Chicago
Temple, while Joey was hunting for some material with which
to make molds. IW thought that Joey had a pretty healthy
give and take relationship with his mother. He did not have
a need to play up to IW or to impress her, but more or less
ignored IW, and went about making the usual demands for
soda pop, some new toys and something more entertaining to
do than just sit while mother was in an interview.

IW arranged with mother for temorary plans regarding/pre-
placement visit at LB and final placement, not mentioning
dates but just giving a general picture of the procedure.

IW cleared certain legal technicalities regarding the
Blakemore intake on this date, Mrs. Duncan will confirm
these in a letter to IW, also enclosing the court decree
for L.B. review prior to the placement. Mrs. Duncan
stated that at the end of each month, L.B. should take
the initiative in sending in a claim blank for the total
amount due L.B. for the care of the Blakemore children.

J. T. Blakemore

This claim blank should arrive at the Du Page county court office by the end of the month for which the payment is due. Mrs. Duncan will send some claim blanks in her letter to IW.

Mrs. Duncan stated definitely that IW will not need to appear at a court hearing. It was learned that Mr. William Guild handled the dependency hearing. He is State's Attorney for Du Page county. The judge who heard the case was Russell W. Keeney. He took a keen interest in Mrs. Blakemore's situation. He felt that she was a very worthy mother - who needed the help of their court in working out adequate plans for her children. He felt that it was important that the court give this mother a great deal of support so that she might keep her children in a close relationship with her. The P.O. goes by the name of Mrs. Pearl A. Duncan.

Du Page court will be responsible to L.B. for the total amount of $95.00 monthly for both children, unless they re-open the financial arrangement with L.B. and they and L.B. together should decide on some different financial agreement. IW left it that Mrs. Duncan would feel free to discuss a different financial plan with L.B. if she felt this was indicated and, in turn, L.B. could take the same approach.

Mrs. Duncan felt that it was a pleasure to work with the kind of a situation where she felt that the children were being helped at an early stage and were not left until serious personality problems had developed. She called the Blakemore children "dependent children" and although there was a definite commitment when the case was first heard by Judge Keeney, it is considered a court hearing concerning a dependency situation. Mrs. Duncan seemed very cooperative in her entire attitude toward L.B.'s intake study and final court arrangements. She did state that since their court had no emergency placement service that they often could not make use of institutions who would make long intake studies, because placement was needed prior to the time that the intake study could be concluded. IW discussed in brief the intake study at L.B. Mrs. Duncan appeared interested in this and also asked regarding our general intake situation. She felt she might want to refer some children to us at some future time. IW commented to her that Mrs. Blakemore had felt it a pleasant experience to appear at Du Page county court and expressed the appreciation of L.B. for this kind of situation. IW will clear with Mrs. Duncan when a definite placement date is set and Mrs. Duncan will arrange this change on the court commitment papers.   *ce*

The decree for divorce listed Ruth Blakemore as plaintiff and Donald Blakemore as defendent. The number is 46-1095. Mark Bemis was Mrs. Blakemore's attorney. The decree listed Mrs. B. as a resident of Du Page county and charged that the defendent was guilty of adultery. Mrs. B. was awarded sole care and custody of the two children and was stated as being entitled to receive alimony. The court decree ordered that the court should retain jurisdiction of the parties involved for the purpose of awarding to mother a reasonable sum of money for her alimony and child support money for the minor

NAME: BLAKEMORE   PAGE: 18

children. The divorce was granted January 10, 1947 by Judge
Win G. Knoch.

IW reviewed the marriage license of Donald Blakemore and Ruth
Barnes, married December 21, 1936 in Corydon, Iowa.

IW saw the second marriage certificate of Donald and Ruth B.
The marriage took place January 27, 1948, in Camden County,
Georgia.   CE:ev

Medical blanks received by L.B. and later given to the
hospital for their records.   CE:ev

Received letter from Du Page county court enclosing commitment
papers.   CE:ev
Pre-placement Conference.
Mrs. Blakemore brought her two children to LB on this date
for the pre-placement visit, arranged previously by IW. After
IW introduced Mrs. B. to Mr. Gale, case worker, and introduced
Mr. Gale to the two Blakemore children, IW and Mrs. B. spent
a short time discussing additional social history which was
needed for the completion of IW's study.

When mother separated from her husband, she was living with
her mother-in-law at the time and the children were with her.
Following her divorce, mother placed Joey with a maternal
aunt, Mrs. Wineinger, in Dexter, Iowa, during the summer of
1947. At the same time, Judy went to live with Mr. and Mrs.
Roach. Mr. Roach was mother's employer at the time. When
the maternal aunt felt that she was unable to keep Joey through
the school year, mother learned of the Engstrom Home through
her employer, Mr. Roach, and placed Joey in this home in the
fall of 1947.

Engstrom Home consists of Vernon and Pauline Engstrom and a seventeen year old daughter, Mary Joe. They live at 12 Mohawk Drive,
Blackhawk Heights, Clarendon Hills, Illinois, telephone Hinsdale
526 J. Mother feels that Mrs. Engstrom was under the impression
that she might be able to convince Mrs. Blakemore to place Joey
for adoption when mother made the private foster home placement.

At the same time Joey was being placed in the Engstrom Home,
mother felt that Judy was not too satisfactorily placed with the
Roaches since Mrs. Roach worked a good deal of the time in the
same restaurant in which mother worked, and Judy had to be at the
restaurant with mother some of the time. Mother went to the home

5. My father was twenty-one when he married my
   mother, and yet he had been married before and had
   had a child. I was told that that marriage was annulled.
   I've never met my half sister. They say her name is
   Barbara and that she is now a big editor or publisher in
   New York City. I can't even begin to imagine how to
   find her, assuming she would want to be found, but I
   wish her well.

235

of Rev. Devore in hopes of talking to Rev. Devore about a
person he might know who would take Judy. Rev. Devore
wasn't home so mother learned through Mrs. Devore of the
Bradford home. Judy went to live in this home in the fall
of 1947 and remained in the Bradford home until Mrs. Bradford
needed to have an operation in the spring of 1948. It was at
this time, Judy went to live with the Engstroms. Engstroms
had been thinking in terms of having Judy with them for some
time. Both children remained in the Engstrom Home until August
of 1948. At this time, Mrs. Engstrom felt that she couldn't
keep the children any longer unless she was able to adopt them,
and so mother needed to make other plans. For the time being,
she took the children to live with her, and she was living in
the private home of Mr. and Mrs. Henning in Downers Grove. This
placement did not work out very satisfactorily since Mrs. Henning
had children of her own and a total of five children was too much
for her to care for. In January of 1949, mother was very discouraged about trying to find proper homes for her two children.
She went back to Iowa in order to be closer to her parents. She
had the children with her in Des Moines, Iowa and lived in a
place that was designed to provide residence for working mothers
and provide someone to care for the children while the mother worked.
Mother worked at this time but wasn't ready to handle the financial
expense of this plan. She stayed in Des Moines only ten weeks.
In the meantime, the Engstroms had been writing to her that they
would like to have her come back to Illinois, and the Engstroms
indicated a willingness to take the children back.

In March of 1949, the children went back into the Engstrom Home
and mother went back to work at her old place. They stayed until
August of 1950 at which time Mrs. Engstrom again requested removal
of the children because she felt that she couldn't keep them
any longer unless she was able to adopt them. Mother felt that
perhaps she was trying to put her under pressure to place the
children for adoption, but Mother frankly indicated she is
not certain about that observation, however. It was in August of
1950 that mother called L.B. about the possibility of placement.
See back dictation in this case record.

In August of 1950, Judy went to live with Mr. and Mrs. W. T.
McDonell, 4922 Saratoga, Downers Grove, Illinois. Mrs. McDonell
was described as being a pretty adequate foster mother. Mrs. M.
is interested in boarding children on a foster home basis from an
agency and may possibly contact us. Mother thought at the present
time, Mrs. McDonell was pretty absorbed in caring for an aged
mother and also some relatives had moved into the home. But should
this situation change, mother feels Mrs. McDonell would make a
good foster mother. Judy was removed from the McDonell home when
Mrs. McDonell was too tied up with the care of her aged mother.
Judy then went to live with Mr. and Mrs. Carl Lang, 6030 S. Bentley,
Clarendon Hills, Illinois. She is, at present, in this home.

In August of 1950, Jody went to live with his paternal uncle and
has been there up until the last few weeks, from which time he has
been camping around with various friends of his.

NAME: BLAKEMORE   PAGE: 20

Mother feels that the children, as a whole, have had fairly
good foster home placements but she is quite concerned about
the many moves they've had and feels it is about time they
are establishing a home base. Mother brought this feeling
out to *Intake* Worker as well as to Mr. Gale during her
first meeting with him at the beginning of the pre-placement
visit.

Joey knew that Mother re-married her husband in January of
1948. Judy found out about it later, although Mother had not
told her. They also know some of the reasons why mother has
separated from her husband. Mother has described this
mostly to the children on the basis that her husband continued
to move around *and* not establish a home for them, did not
support them adequately during the period of being separated
from them and in general *did* not *show* much interest in
family life.

Intake worker indicated that she would not be seeing mother
again excepting in casual meetings on the campus and that
Mr. Gale would be continuing to work with her. This had
previously been discussed with mother also.

                                              CE:ev

Mrs. Blakemore and the two children made a pre-placement visit
to LBO on 8-15-51. The children were placed on 8-17-51. They
came as wards of the Du Page County Court and under the guardianship of LBO. In placing the children, Mrs. Blakemore had spoken
of their needing care until they were old enough to be able to
live with her without supervision while she was working. These
plans have not been referred to except on one occasion on 1-28-52,
when Mrs. Blakemore commented on how excellent she felt the children had adjusted to LBO, and she hoped that they would be able
to continue to stay there. The case worker agreed that they had
been doing very well but pointed up some of the disadvantages
of continued institutional care and indicated that some of these
might be remedied by boarding home care. Mrs. Blakemore expressed
concern with regard to the experiences she had had during the
children's placement with Mr. and Mrs. Engstrom, the couple that
had become so attached to the children that they wished to adopt
them. The CW agreed that this was indeed a disadvantage, that if
such a plan were considered desirable, a couple would need to be
found who understood the close relationship between the children
and their mother and that this would continue to be fostered wit.
no hope of adoption.

For the first month, Mrs. Blakemore visited the children each
week on her one day off, but by that time realized that she was

J. T. Blakemore

not able to continue with this plan as it required from six to
eight hours of traveling in order for her to do this and with
only one day off, it did not leave her with sufficient time to
take care of her own needs. Since October 1st, she had visited bi-
weekly, was able to have the children visit with her and friends
for one week at Christmas time. Mrs. B. is a mother who is warm
and understanding, who, over a period of six years, has adjusted
herself to thinking in terms of the best interest of the children,
as being in placement away from herself. She has a light sense
of humor, and though maintaining high standards for her children,
is able to give them considerable freedom within this relationship.
When the worker visited her at her home on 8-16-51, prior to the
children's placement, she continued her work as they talked together, the children helping her pack. She directed them occasionally with about fifty percent effectiveness and did not
seem overly concerned that they did not immediately respond to her
demands. After the children's placement, Mrs. Blakemore seemed
realistically accepting of the fact that the children would have
to work through their problems of adjustment in their new groups,,
and that this could be expected to take some time. She said she
would give sympathy and encouragement, but would also indicate
that these were things that they needed to help themselves with.
She feels that whenever the children have problems that they consider to be really serious, they will discuss them with her and
she feels that the children have come to make excellent adjustment
since the time of their placement at LBO. Mrs. Blakemore has been
excellent in her cooperation with LBO and has always fulfilled her
commitments to make visits, keep appointments, pay bills. On one
occasion before giving Judy some used clothes that were in good
condition, she discussed this first with the worker, explaining
that Joey had been accustomed to receiving this before and enjoyed
having it despite its used condition. She asked, however, if this
was all right with LBO and was told that it was.

In addition to her regular board payments of $95.00 per month,
for the two children, Mrs. Blakemore has been able to provide for
some of the additional expenses of the children. These include
$12.35 for Judy's glasses and more recently she has been paying
toward the hospital bill incurred at the time of Joey's appendectomy. She had indicated that she would be willing to try to meet
the added expense of Joey's camp period this summer, but following
Joey's appendectomy, it was decided that she should devote her
resources to paying this bill and that LBO would assume the expense for Joey's camp. The hospital bill amounted to $127.80.
Mrs. Blakemore felt that she could pay $10.00 every two weeks and
on 4/21, 5/5, and 5/19, paid $10.00 on each date. She was not able
to make a payment on 6/2/52, however. Mrs. Blakemore has not had
any form of Health Insurance and has said she has not been able to
discover a policy that she could be sure was a good one. She has
said that a company she is familiar with is trying to bring out a
policy in June and she hopes to be able to make arrangements for
this at that time.

Joey is seen as a likeable, good-looking boy who is able to relate

NAME: BLAKEMORE   PAGE: 22

satisfactorily to adults. He is reserved and gives the appearance
of being a little shy at first, but seemed able to indicate his
true feelings with some depth. Joey seemed able to accept the
case worker readily at their first meeting and asked many questions
concerning LBO's activities, kids, and where they would live.
Joey showed a natural amount of anxiety as he met his houseparents
and boys with whom he was to live. He later told the case worker
that he was worried about the initiation the boys told him he would
receive. Although Joey was placed in the older boys' unit, he
would be nine months younger than any other child there. With
respect to his being sensitive about his being a year behind at
school, it was pointed out to him that there were four other
children in the same circumstances. Joey has revealed an ability
to meet many of his own problems and appears to have made a very
satisfactory adjustment. His housefather said that he felt that
Joey was rather babyish when he first knew him, but that he had
shown much improvement during his placement. He said that Joey
had cried a lot when he first came, and though this continued to
be true to a certain extent, it was not as much as it had been.
Joey's main problem when he first arrived was his concern over
the other children picking on him. He said he was trying hard to
make friends with one of the older boys who was doing this, and
though occasionally he thought he would like to be transferred to
the youngest children's living unit, he had decided that he would
make a go of it with the older boys. By the middle of September
he was commenting favorably on the adults responsible for his car
and said that while the kids still picked on him sometimes, he
thought he could take care of it. By the middle of October, Mrs.
Blakemore said that he no longer had any complaints to tell her of,
and that he generally felt that LBO was a swell place. Joey was
very upset when late in October it was discovered that he had been
in the company of another boy at the time the other boy had stolen
some luminous paint. The boy had apparently given a can to Joey
so that he would not tell of this. Joey had apparently not wanted
to inform on the other child's activity and had thereby become a
party to the theft himself. Joey cried and became almost physically
sick over his concern as to what his mother would think of it.
Joey has in no way been associated with any thefts since that time.
Joey is still thought of as the youngest member of his group and is
not looked up to as a leading participant in it, but he plays with
many of the children and enters into group activities. He is fairly
clean in his room and in his person and is able to do his jobs about
the Hall well.

Joey appears to have a very excellent relationship with his mother
and to have a great deal of affection for her. He seems to be able
to discuss problems with her and looks forward to and enjoys her
visits. Joey also appears to have a very good relationship with
his sister. At the time of the pre-placement visit, Judy said she
would come to play with her brother all the time. Joey responded
good-naturedly by saying, "No, you won't. I'm a boy and you're a
girl." To which Judy replied, "No, I'm a boy - tom-boy!" The
children, however, do play together frequently and seem to get along
well. During the first part of her placement, Judy had a very
difficult time relating to the other girls and Joey expressed considerable concern over this. He told the case worker that she came

6. I don't remember a thing about this luminous paint
   incident, but I'm not at all surprised that I cried and
   was scared about my mother finding out about it. I
   remember once stealing a piece of candy and feeling
   so guilty about it that I told on myself. I knew then that
   I'd never be a thief.

J. T. Blakemore

and talked to him about the problems she was having, and Joey
was very troubled that he was not able to help his sister.
Joey was helped to understand that Judy's houseparents would
help her as much as they could, and that the case worker would
be helping her also, which seemed to relieve his anxiety, somewhat.

Joey has averaged about a C- in his school work, but this is
ranged all the way from B's down to F's, history and science
being his too best subjects and arithmetic and spelling being
the subjects in which he receives F's. He has received very
poor grades under social attitudes, however, and this may well
have had considerable affect on his academic grades, and in his
next to the last marking period, he received all Unsatisfactories
but in his final grading, he only received an Unsatisfactory in
self-control and self-reliance and was given a grade of Superior
for responsibility. Mrs. Whitaker, Education Director, believed
that Joey's reaction to his teacher was due largely to the teacher's
personality and is not necessarily a reflection on Joey.

Joey's health has been excellent during this period and the only
activity in this area has been an appendectomy at Lake Forest
Hospital on 3-31-52. Joey made an excellent recovery and returned
to LB on 4-6-52 and to school on 4-7-52.

Judy is a friendly, outgoing youngster who appears to relate
superficially with adults . Although she has been able to
discuss some of her problems with her mother and brother, it
has been hard for her todo so with the houseparents and case
worker. Her houseparents believe, however, that it is
helpful to her to discuss these problems as they arise, as
she seems to benefit from talking them over. Judy has generally
been able to relate to adults more readily than to the other
children. Although her problems have generally been centered
around her contemporaries, she was able to express hostility
toward her housefather, to her mother, on 10-22-51. Two weeks
later she remarked, however, that while the housefather was
grumpy, he was okay. It has been very hard for a houseparent
to accept her at times, however, because of what appears to
be a deceitful attitude. She will agree with her houseparents
whenever they are disciplining another child and give the appearance of wanting to conform when they are talking with her. Her
behavior is not consistent with this during their absence, however,
Recently, however, Mr. and Mrs. Forsberg feel that Judy has been
more consistent in her behavior and that, while not demanding, she
really wants to be accepted by her houseparents. Judy's greatest
problems have been in her relationships with the other children.
Although she was gravely concerned about their not liking her,
she assumed a role of complete independence. The children, at
first, reacted strongly against her fine appearance and her good
clothes. Judy was acutely aware of this and complained of it
to her case worker. She was not able, however, to consider how
she might alter this situation but instead wanted her case worker
to in some way make the other children like her. As a reaction

NAME: BLAKEMORE   PAGE: 24

to this, Judy appeared even more aloof and superior to the
other children and they continued to resent this very much.
Judy said that she knew one of the reasons why she was better
than the other children. This was because her hair was longer
and prettier, and she said defiantly that she was never going
to cut it. After about ten days at LBO, she was able to play
with some of the children one at a time. When she tried to mix
in with group activities, the girls would not accept her. It
was suggested that the houseparents attempt to foster these
individual relationships before she was encouraged to mix with
the group. After about two weeks of placement, the girls seemed
to be a little friendlier toward Judy and she agreed that they
did not pick on her as much. By the middle of October, Mrs.
Blakemore said that Judy still had many gripes but had said
that she would get to like it for her mother. She seemed to
be getting along very well and was occasionally on good terms
with the leader of her Hall group. When there were occasional
differences, Judy would frequently oppose this leader and the
other girls would give in to her. Judy has assumed considerable
status in the group through these means, but did not develop
close friendships as she frequently tattled on the other children
in order to maintain her friendship with the group. There have been
gradual improvements in all of these areas, however, and by February, Judy was playing much more as a part of the group and was
generally liked by the other children. There are occasional
periods when Judy asserts her independence from the entire group
and is rejected by them. This quickly passes, however, and she
is more and more accepted by the children. She usually likes to
play with only one or two other children, however, where she can
usually retain considerable control. She likes dressing up and
roller skating and she is able to engage in healthy, active play
without concern for her appearance or for the play being too rough.
She has had no difficulty in accepting her need to wear glasses
and usually keeps them on at all times.

Judy also seems to have a close relationship with her mother and
seems to look forward to and clearly enjoy their visits. During
the early part of her placement, she was able to discuss with
her mother the various problems that were arising, but at all
times seemed to understand that she must make the best of her
situation at Lake Bluff. Judy usually boasts of the visits with
her mother and tells the other children of the dinners that they
have together and the frequencies of their visits. She has mentioned her father on only one occasion at which time she told
her housemother that her father had left she and her mother alone.
As has been indicated above, Judy appears to have a good relationship with her brother also, and frequently seeks him out as her
protector.

Judy's school adjustment has been generally satisfactory with bot
her behavior and her academic accomplishment considered to be
average.

Judy's health has been very good during this period. Glasses were
prescribed for her on October 20, 1951, and she has been able to
accept the need for wearing them very well.

NAME: BLAKEMORE   PAGE: 25

The last time future plans for these children were discussed
with Mrs. Blakemore, she indicated that she would prefer
continued institutional care, but it seems possible that if
further interpretation is given her concerning the type of
foster home desirable in this situation, that she would be
able to accept boarding home care. She would need to be
helped to an understanding of the advantages of this type
of care, and to be given some assurance that she would not
be threatened by foster parents trying to take her children
from her. Both children seemed to be profiting from institutional care and boarding-home care is not immediately
necessary although Joey would seem ready at this time to make
good use of such care. As Judy is becoming more secure within
her group, she is having less need to defensively assert her
independence, which is of course is not a true independence
at all. Institutional care is also serving to broaden her
sense of values and to relieve her of the need of always
playing the role of a little doll for the benefit of adults.
The strong relationship that exists between these chi ren
is a factor to be considered when boarding home pl ement
is made.

JQG:ev

Mrs. Blakemore visited on 6/16 and 6/30/52. She paid a total
of $30.00 toward Joey's hospital bill reducing the balance
owed to $67.80. When she has completed paying this bill, she
would like to begin paying toward the $55.00 needed to cover
Joey's camp expenses. It was suggested that this might be
difficult for her in addition to the hospital bill, but she said she
would pay it.

Mrs. B. said she would plan to continue visiting on alternate
Mondays at 4:00PM through the Summer unless she requested otherwise. She will have her vacation from 8/1 to 8/16 and may plan
some activity for the children prior to Joey's going to camp
from 8/10 to 8/24.

CASE TRANSFERRED, THIS DATE, TO MRS. CAROL HINDS, C.W. SUPER-
VISOR.

JQG:jcg

NAME: BLAKEMORE   PAGE 26

Present casework assignment was made 11-1-52. See the
social information prepared for Dr. Beiser for psychiatric
consultation 3-26-53.

The mother continues her former employment and maintains
regular bi-weekly visiting with the children. There have
been no changes in plans by the mother for future care and
she would like both children to remain in the institution
indefinitly. Discussion during this period has been concerned with Judy's adjustment in the institution and Joey's
medical problem. In addition to the regular visits to the
institution the children were able to spend Thanksgiving
and Christmas with the mother by staying in homes of her
friends. There was a four day visit at Thanksgiving and
the children spent fifteen days with the mother at Christmas
1952.

Joey has continued to get along well with the boys in his
unit and generally with the children in the institution.
Joey's chief concern has been his disturbance because Judy
has had difficulty with the other children.

Joey is currently enrolled in the fifth grade at the Lake
Bluff Public School where his school progress has been
average in all instances and there are several grades of
good and superior. His school behavior has been satisfactory though he has complained to the house mother that
his teacher is unfair to him.

Joey has been in good health since his appendectomy in
March 1952 until he had what was reported as "fainting
spells" at school on January 15 and 16, 1953. A blood
count revealed that his hemoglobin was very low. He
received iron capsules and a hemoglobic count on 2-18-53
was 77 % as compared to 50% 1-16-53.

NAME: BLAKEMORE   PAGE: 27

PSYCHIATRIC CONSULTATION
3-26-53

Staff members present: Mrs. Hinds, Miss Blunt, Mr. Sumner, Mr. Falby, Mr. Clements, Mr. and Mrs. Bather, Mrs. Harrison, Miss Seemann and Dr. Gross, Clinical Psychologist at Downey.

After review of the case material, Dr. Beiser commented that neither child eats well for an unknown reason, but it appears that they may want the institution to feel bad that they don't eat here. It seems that everything the mother does is right while the institution is always wrong. There is question as to whether mother produces outside influence which would affect Judy's adjustment in the institution. Most children idealize parents and displace hostile feeling they have toward parents to the agency. Such displacement gives hope for the future but makes difficulty in placing reality problems.

Dr. Beiser commented further that these children are not very disorganized but they are more neurotic than many children in our care. Judy will possibly grow up, have many masochistic needs and be a poor, deprived, abused woman. She uses this technique now as a valuable weapon to get punishment. Her guilt apparently catches up with her when others are good to her. Her relationship with Darlene fulfills Darlene's desire to manipulate and Judy's desire to be babied. Her masochistic needs are not complete and her good appearance indicates only partial involvement.

It was suggested that Judy would probably get along better in a foster home but there are dangers that she also idealizes foster home care. Considerable casework service would have to be accomplished with the mother in order to accept foster home care. Judy seems to have need for a simpler environment with fewer activities than afforded in group care. The mother will have to examine her relationship and break certain parts of it in order to free Judy for a satisfactory foster home placement. The agency is justified in saying to the mother that institutional care is harming Judy. It was recognized that mothers need to feel that they are competent and it might be possible to use Mrs. Blakemore's strong feeling of obligation in helping her accept better care for Judy. The psychiatrist felt that mother has a need which is more than to prove she is as a mother but it is as yet unknown. This is indicated by the strong interplay to cause the present neurotic development of these children. The food and eating difficulties may be related to the business of the parent, but this is only speculation.

In response to questions by the housemother as to how she can deal with present behavior, Dr. Beiser stated that housemother can point out to Judy in her times of difficulty that she does not seem to enjoy herself when other children do, and when she should.

MWW:ev   Mirl W. Whitaker,
5/8/53   Caseworker

7. They quote the psychiatrist as saying "Judy will possibly grow up to have many masochistic needs and be a poor, deprived, abused woman." What a shocking, arrogant, unprofessional and cruel thing to put in a report. I can't imagine a psychiatrist doing that today. At least I hope they wouldn't. It sounds like he basically gave up on my sister. He didn't make such harsh, sweeping comments about me, probably because I was a boy. Back then it was fairly common to write off a girl, I suppose. I remember my mother laughing at this quote. She thought Judy would be a movie star. She told Judy, "You're not like that and

NAME: BLAKEMORE   PAGE: 28

During this period the mother has continued to visit on
alternate Mondays but does not like to talk with worker.
She was seen for an office interview on 3-30-53. At that
time, mother was informed that Judy's behavior was essentially
the same though Mother finds it difficult to see any problem
with this. Mother is hopeful that improvement will come and
does not want to consider other planning. Worker suggested
that agency feels Judy is not being helped in the institution
and we would like to discuss other kinds of care for her
daughter. Mother does not want to consider separation of the
children and inasmuch as agency does not have foster home
services available at this time the matter was not pressed
further.

The worker had a personal interview with Miss Sorenson 4-1-53,
Judith's present teacher in the Lake Bluff School. She commented that Joey was in her class last year and at first he
was very interested in school work and had a keen desire to
participate and was generally a good student. After a few
weeks, his attitude changed, he lost interest and his whole
personality seemed to be dulled by institutional care. Instead of continuing to make progress, Miss Sorenson reported
that Joey actually "went backwards".

In discussing Judy's present school adjustment, it was revealed that she had been tardy twelve times during the current
school year and is "not getting anywhere in school". She
prefers to sit at her desk and not move away for any class or
group participation. Judy squints through her glasses and
asks the teacher to repeat though the teacher is aware that
she has no hearing difficulty. Judy can spell but insists that
she is unable to do so. Her school achievement is very, very
poor at the present time. She has been placed in the slowest
reading class and is now the slowest one in the slow group.
A current school achievement test showed that she earned 3.4
when average achievement should have been 4.6.

Aside from the convenience to the mother, little can be said
in favor of continued institutional care for these children,
particularly Judy. It is becoming more and more obvious that
not only are they not being helped but are actually being
damaged by continued institutional stay. Judy's behavior has
been more symptomatic but Joey also resorts to frequent "tattling"
and gets into difficulty with several of the boys. The worker
has been unsuccessful in helping the mother to accept her children's reaction to institutional care as she insists that it
offers much more stability than they ever had previously. The
agency will need to decide how long they can continue institutional care for the children and when it will be necessary to
insist with the mother that other plans be made.

THIS CASE TRANSFERRED TO MR. ANGUS SUMNER, CASEWORKER, 5-6-53.
                                                    MWW:ev

you're not gonna turn out like that." After that, we all
considered it to be water under the bridge and we
moved on. So were that doctor's predictions about
Judy true? She definitely had a harder time during our
childhood. She has known deprivation and abuse. She
is not what you'd consider wealthy, but she owns her
own home. And through it all, she has been happy-go-
lucky. My mother used to say, "Judy gets over
everything just like that, but Joe doesn't." Is it real, or
a coping mechanism? I don't know. But I applaud her
for having overcome so much. We're still very close.

<u>CONFERENCE WITH DR. BEISER</u>
<u>March 26, 1953</u>

CHILD: Judy Lynn Blakemore, born 10-22-43
                         LBO Placement: 8-17-51

REASON FOR REFERRAL: Discussion of present behavior in
                     the institution setting and assis-
                     tance in planning for future care.

Conference with Dr. Beiser, re Judy Blakemore, March 26, 1953
- -

IDENTIFYING INFORMATION

Father: Donald A. Blakemore, born 9-20-15; occupation: chef;
address unknown

Mother: Ruth Barnes, born 2-14-16; occupation: waitress;
address: Westmont, Illinois

The parents were married 12-21-36, divorced 1-10-47,
remarried 1-27-48.

Children:
Joseph Thomas, born 7-1-41; LBO Placement, 8-17-51
Judy Lynn, born 10-22-43; LBO Placement, 8-17-51

The father has never been seen by any member of the agency
staff. All information available about him has been given
by the mother. He was born in Iowa, completed two years of
high school, has no military record, and his only employment
has been that as a chef. The father has seen neither of the
children since before the divorce in January 1947. The father
was married once prior to marriage to mother and had one
child by the former marriage. During the early part of his
marriage to mother, father paid $2.50 weekly for support of
the first child, but discontinued when his former wife remarried. Following marriage to mother, the parents moved all
over the country. Father would work a short while and then
move. Mother talked about this tendency of her husband to
move about the country as his chief negative so far as being
a good husband and father. She felt that some men drank and
some men move around. "A chef does one or the other." Mother
wanted to have children and settle down, but father never
agreed to this, except on real insistence from mother. Following birth of the children, he supported the family well for the
first few years, but he seemed to act to them more as an older
brother rather than as a father. He was quite immature in his
ways; though he seemed to like his home, he could not stay in
one place. After birth of the second child, the parents purchased a home in Round Lake while the father was working in
Chicago. He first came home on week-ends and sometimes during
the week, but his visits became less and less frequent. The
father maintained relationships with other women at this time
but mother feels that separation was primarily due to his inability to assume responsibility for his family rather than
interference by other persons.

Mother is one of four children who was born and reared in a
small Iowa town. Following graduation from high school, she
worked as a telephone operator for two years. After this,
in company with some girl friends, she moved to Des Moines,
and began working in a restaurant. It was at this time that
she met her husband.

Conference with Dr. Beiser, re Judy Blakemore, March 26, 1953
- -

Mother has been described variously by differing workers.
Intake worker described her as being "dressed very attractively" and "she makes a very good appearance". After placement she was described as "a mother who is warm and understanding, who over a period of six years has adjusted herself
to thinking in terms of the best interest of the children
in being in placement away from herself." She "has been excellent in her cooperation with Lake Bluff Orphanage and has
always fulfilled her commitments to make visits, keep appointments and pay bills."

The experience of the present worker with mother has found her
to be an intelligent but evasive person in terms of discussing
institutional placement realistically. Mother gives the impression of having been considerably burdened by the care of
these children and being quite pleased that their basic physical needs can be met in an institution without thought for
change. She is able to respond to incidental requests and discussion about the care of the children, but any thought or
suggestion that another type of care might be desirable, brings
an immediate evasiveness and resistance from the mother. She
has maintained visits regularly, kept her promises adequately
to the children, fulfilled the budgeted financial responsibili-
ties, and complies with requests concerning routine institutional care.

There has not been an opportunity to see mother with the children
except for very brief periods of time. She takes them away from
the institution for an evening meal when she is able to visit on
alternate Mondays. This contact and outing has been of considerable value to both children and the mother seems to realize the
opportunity to eat the meal away provides considerable pleasure
for the children. The mother is not demanding of the children
and seems interested in them but the worker has not observed attitudes or behavior which would be characterized as "warm".

During intake interview, mother stated that Judy was cute and
everybody knew it. She showed considerable pride in talking
about her daughter, but felt that Judy should be given a more
realistic picture of how to get along with people. Mother wanted
Judy to be helped so that she does not use her looks in attempting
to get things from adults. Mother felt that Judy had certain resentments against being petted by adults, but the intake worker
felt that Judy really enjoyed this sort of attention. Mother
felt that people had always thought Judy was very attractive and
given her too much attention. When intake worker suggested that
Judy might find it difficult to share with other children in the
institution and particularly to share adult leaders, the mother
responded by saying she felt the children had been spoiled by
their various foster parents. Mother said Judy is able "to work"
adults and has been allowed to do this. Mother wanted these
behavior patterns "broken down somewhat". Intake worker quoted
"Mother is not punitive, at least not too obviously, in their
attitude concerning the value of institutional placement for her
children, but actually is quite able to see desirable values in

Conference with Dr. Beiser, re Judy Blakemore, March 26, 1953
- -

such a placement, and understand how a group setting can contribute to the growth of the children." It was suspected that
the children may have demanded "too much from this mother and
she really felt as though she spoiled them". Mother, on one
occasion described Judy as "being fussy about her clothes".

Mother notes that the relationship between herself and father
became particularly more difficult following the birth of Judy.
The relationship which this child had with her father is relatively unknown, but mother stated that while Joey "grew close
to his father, Judy took a more negative attitude toward him."
She would often resent the father being around and would hold
off her father so that he could not get too close to her. This
reportedly hurt the father quite a bit. Judy has not seen the
father since she was three years of age. At the time of placement, the mother apparently discussed the causes for divorce
with the children but we do not now know Judy's feeling about
her father. Joey knew that mother remarried father in January
1948, and though Judy was not told about it, she later discovered this fact. Her reaction to this discovery is unknown.

Before placement, Judy completed the first two grades of school
and had kindergarten prior to first grade work. Her school a-
chievement prior to placement was better than a B average. She
was well liked by the teachers and had no difficulty with
adequate school progress.

All placements prior to Judy's acceptance for institutional
care, 8-17-51, by LBO, were made privately by the mother.
Both children stayed with the mother following the divorce
until the summer of 1947 when Judy was placed with the family
of mother's employer. This placement was discontinued in
the fall of 1947 because the foster mother worked. The second
placement lasted from the fall of 1947 to the spring of 1948
and was terminated because the foster mother had to be hospitalized for surgery. The third placement was made for the first
time in a family where Joey was also present. This placement
lasted from the spring of 1948 to the fall of 1948 and was
terminated because of foster parents' insistance upon adoption
if the children were to remain in the family. The mother removed the children and kept them with herself for a period of
time in Illinois and then returned to her home state of Iowa.
The financial pressures upon the mother made the continuation
of this plan unfeasible and in March of 1949, both children returned to the family where they had been last placed. This
fourth placement lasted until August of 1950 when the foster
parents again were pressing for adoption. The children were
again removed and from August of 1950 to the spring of 1951,
Judy was again placed alone in a family where care was terminated
because the foster mother had to give care to her own mother.
The sixth placement was made in the spring of 1951 and continued
until August when Judy came to Lake Bluff Orphanage. With the
exception of the mother's brief living experience in Iowa, Judy
has lived in a relatively small geographical area in a suburb
southwest of Chicago during this entire time. The replacement
from home to home did not always mean a change in schools.

Conference with Dr. Beiser, re Judy Blakemore, March 26, 1953
- -

Information for Judy's adjustment from the time of placement until July 1952 comes from the recording of the worker assigned to the case during that period.

Judy is a friendly outgoing youngster who appears to relate superficially with adults. Although she has been able to discuss some of her problems with her mother and brother, it has been hard for her to do so with the houseparents and caseworker. Her problems have generally centered around her peers but she was able to express hostility against the housefather as her mother in the fall of 1951. It has been difficult for houseparent staff to accept Judy at times because of what appears to them to be "a deceitful attitude". Judy appears to be accepting and understanding of requests during discussions with her but her behavior is not consistent during the houseparents' absence. Upon arrival, Judy was concerned that the other children did not like her and reacted by assuming a role of complete independence. The other children reacted strongly against her fine appearance and her good clothes. Judy was aware of this and complained to her case worker. She was unable to consider how she might alter the situation but instead wanted her caseworker to make the other children like her. As a reaction, Judy appeared more aloof and superior to the other children and they continued their resentment toward her. Judy told case worker that one of the reasons why she was better than the other children was because her hair was longer and prettier and she defiantly stated she would never cut it.

After ten days of placement, Judy was able to play with some of the children one at a time. The girls, as a group, would not accept her into their activities. At the end of two weeks, Judy stated that the girls "do not pick on me as much". The mother reported to case worker two months later that Judy still had many gripes but had said she would begin to like the institution for her mother's sake. Judy began to get along better with Darlene Brooks who has assumed considerable leadership toward group activities. Judy never hesitated from the first to oppose Darlene when the occasion arose and this won Judy status with the other children who were frightened of Darlene. Judy did not develop close friendships, however, as she frequently tattled on the other children. It was reported in February 1953 that Judy was playing much more as a part of the group and was generally liked by the other children. There still were occasional periods when Judy asserted her independence from the entire group and was rejected by them. These periods of independence have grown shorter and shorter in length. She still liked to play with only one or two children at a time where she could retain considerable control. She is able to roller skate and engage in healthy, active play without concern for her appearance or for the play being too rough.

Information from the first ten months of institutional placement indicate that Judy seemed to have a close relationship with her mother and looked forward to and enjoyed their visits. She has used the visits partly to discuss the problems which

Conference with Dr. Beiser, re Judy Blakemore, March 26, 1953
- -
page six

she found in the institution, but at all times, seemed to understand that "she must make the best of her situation at Lake Bluff".
Judy usually boasts of the dinners with her mother and tells other
children what she eats during the visit. She has mentioned her
father on only one occasion at which time she told her housemother
that her father had left her and her mother alone.

During the early part of placement when Judy was having difficulty
with the other girls, Joey expressed considerable concern about
this to the case worker. He informed case worker that Judy
talked with him about the problems she was having and Joey was
troubled when he was not able to help her. Joey was helped to
understand that Judy's houseparents would help her as much as
they could and that the case worker would be helping her also.
This seemed to relieve his anxiety somewhat.

Judy's school adjustment was reported to have been "generally
satisfactory with both behavior and academic accomplishment
considered to be average".

Judy has been in good health since her admission to agency care.
Classes were prescribed for her October 1951 which she has been
able to accept readily.

The houseparents in the unit where Judy has been living since
admission, left the agency employment August 1, 1952. The
case worker assigned to this family left in July, 1952, and
the present case work assignment was made November 1, 1952.
During the first conference with the houseparents in November
1952, the housemother and the associate reported that Judy was
having many problems in the unit. It was revealed that this
child expects more personal attention from the girls and the
houseparents than the other children. She likes to play "house"
with the other children and always is the baby. She enjoys
being the baby and being treated as one. After the summer vacation, the other children said they wished Judy had not returned.
She cries easily, hangs on the other girls, and complains that
the former houseparents were mean. Judy reports that the mother
says LBO is the best place for her (Judy), but Judy exclaims she
would not think so if she only knew what happened here. The
children continue to see the mother bi-weekly when she comes
after school and takes them out for supper. Usually Judy has
a stomach ache after the mother leaves and after the other girls
are in bed. She then comes to the houseparents' room to complain
of her illness. At other times, Judy has many complaints about
headaches, tooth aches, stomach aches, and other difficulties.
She does not like to assume responsibility for wrongs she has
done. She wants the biggest piece of cake, and the choice in
any selection. For the attitude, the other children frequently
"gang up" on her. She gets along better with the boys than
with the girls and manages to be invited to many birthday parties.
Her appetite is poor, she eats little except for treats, and the
housemother does not believe that Judy can eat as much as she
reports during the visits with her mother. The housemother for
the younger girls reported that Judy had been getting the younger
girls to carry her books to and from school with the promise to
pay them for the service.

8. The way the report reads, the Engstroms DID want to adopt both of us. My mother always said she had to tell the people at Lake Bluff that little white lie so she'd have a better chance of getting us placed in the orphanage. She felt that if she led the authorities to believe that the Engstroms were trying to take both of her children away from her, they'd take us in. She was able to convince them even though, in reality, I had been living with the Engstroms much longer than my sister had.

Conference with Dr. Beiser, re Judy Blakemore, March 26, 1953
- -

The nature of this November report has persisted during subse-
quent months and the only variation seems to be the name of
the child with whom Judy gets into difficulty. In January,
Judy became involved in a fight with Dorothy for which both
girls were sent to their room. Judy left her room, however,
and went to Wadsworth I to get Joey to come back to the unit
and "beat up Dorothy". When the housemother talked with her,
Judy cried and felt very sorry for herself and said that the
mother had told Joey to take care of her. Judy was unable to
accept any responsibility for her own participation in the
affair. Later in the month after what appeared to be a very
pleasant day for Judy, in company with a staff child, she
got into trouble with Beverly at bedtime. She then complained
to the housemother that there are "too many girls here". "They
all gang up on me." She wished that her mother had never heard
of LBO. Judy said that she liked the foster homes and wished
she had never come here.

In February during one meal time, Judy began crying when she
was invited by the other girls at her table to participate in
a game. She later responded by crying to an invitation from
Beverly to read with her. Judy told the housemother there
were too many people here to be happy but it was"okay with one
or two". She cried after returning from a Valentine party
which from all known information she enjoyed. The housemother
reports that in March Judy again left her room after being
sent there by the Associate Housemother following a disturbance
with two of the other girls. When Judy becomes upset, she acts
impulsively and though she gets over it shortly, she has not been
able to accept limitations which are accepted by the other children. Her difficulty has been expanding quantitatively, if not
qualitatively. She is usually discontent when she becomes angry
with one of the girls in her own unit until she has brought this
to the attention of the other girl's older sister. During recent weeks, she has not only had to accept a great deal of hostility and rejection from the children her own age, but also the
girls from the older unit.

There have been two Progress Reports from the Lake Bluff Public
School where Judy is now enrolled in the fourth grade. Her
school achievement is erratic and varies from some very acceptable better-than-average grades to average and unsatisfactory
grades. She has the best achievement in art, physical education,
and penmanship. She appears to be having difficulty in reading,
arithmetic, geography and spelling.

Judy continues to be in good health and has had no significant
illness during this summary period.

The mother has been evasive in discussing Judy's present adjustment with the worker and has played down the symptoms which her
daughter displays. She postponed a case work appointment for
two weeks, stating she was unable to visit, but later did visit
at the scheduled time. After an early discussion of Judy's behavior with case worker, the mother went to the housemother to
learn about Judy's adjustment.

Conference with Dr. Beiser, re Judy Blakemore, March 26, 1953
- -
                                            page eight

The worker has seen mother on two occasions, specifically to
discuss Judy's behavior, and at both times she tried to inter-
pret Judy's difficulties as those of a child new to institution.
The mother thought that Judy was getting along better and stated
that she liked the present houseparents and that the behavior
would probably not continue much longer. Mother showed real
concern that the adjustment of the children is just opposite
from their adjustment prior to institutional care. Joey showed
continual behavior problems prior to institutional care when
he was in a series of foster homes. At that time Judy did not
have any difficulty getting along in the foster homes and her
school achievement was considerably better than at the present
time. The mother wondered if Joey "gives her too much attention".
The mother stated that Judy "will sob if she gets enough attention". It was exceedingly difficult for mother to understand
why "smart kids don't do well at school". The worker expressed
the feeling that Judy probably needed considerably more attention
than she was able to receive in the group setting. It was worker's
feeling that Judy was having progressively more difficulty with
the children and that this behavior was not likely to lessen as
long as she did not receive more individual attention. Worker
thought that it would be well to consider plans for some other
type of care for Judy. The mother is quite fearful about foster
home placement because of the previous experience she had in
making arrangements herself. She hopes that it will be possible
for Judy to remain in institutional care where she can be close
to her brother.

This is an attractive nine-year old girl who can hardly remember
her father and who has received care outside her own family for
the last six years. She got along without noticeable difficulty
during the period 1947 through August 1951, though she experienced
seven moves in different homes during that time. Institutional
placement in August 1951 was marked with disturbance on the part
of the child and resistance and rejection by the peer group.
The rejection by the group appears to have modified during the
first six to eight months of placement, but it has now increased
during recent months. Judy is aggressive, demanding, babyish,
disregarding of wishes by other children, frightened by groups,
evasive of personal responsibility and disappointed with the
attention which she receives from adults.

1) Are there reasons why foster home care should not be planned
   for Judy?

2) Is her present behavior primarily reactive to group living
   or are there deeper emotional needs that would be equally
   unsatisfied in foster home care?

3) If foster home care is decided upon, and pending such placement, are there suggestions or modifications in present care
   which would be helpful to Judy?

MWW:ev
3-20-53

J. T. Blakemore

PSYCHIATRIC CONSULTATION
3-26-53

Staff members present: Mrs. Hinds, Miss Blunt, Mr. Sumner,
Mr. Falby, Mr. Clements, Mr. and Mrs. Bather, Mrs. Harrison,
Miss Seemann and Dr. Gross, Clinical Psychologist at Downey.

After review of the case material, Dr. Beiser commented that
neither child eats well for an unknown reason, but it appears
that they may want the institution to feel bad that they don't
eat here. It seems that everything the mother does is right
while the institution is always wrong. There is question as
to whether mother produces outside influence which would affect Judy's adjustment in the institution. Most children
idealize parents and displace hostile feeling they have toward
parents to the agency. Such displacement gives hope for the
future but makes difficulty in placing reality problems.

Dr. Beiser commented further that these children are not very
disorganized but they are more neurotic than many children in
our care. Judy will possibly grow up, have many masochistic
needs and be a poor, deprived, abused woman. She uses this
technique now as a valuable weapon to get punishment. Her guilt
apparently catches up with her when others are good to her.
Her relationship with Darlene fulfills Darlene's desire to
manipulate and Judy's desire to be babied. Her masochistic
needs are not complete and her good appearance indicates only
partial involvement.

It was suggested that Judy would probably get along better in
a foster home but there are dangers that she also idealizes
foster home care. Considerable casework service would have
to be accomplished with the mother in order to accept foster
home care. Judy seems to have need for a simpler environment
with fewer activities than afforded in group care. The mother
will have to examine her relationship and break certain parts
of it in order to free Judy for a satisfactory foster home
placement. The agency is justified in saying to the mother
that institutional care is harming Judy. It was recognized
that mothers need to feel that they are competent and it
might be possible to use Mrs. Blakemore's strong feeling of
obligation in helping her accept better care for Judy. The
psychiatrist felt that mother has a need which is more than
to prove she is a mother but it is as yet unknown. This is
indicated by the strong interplay to cause the present neurotic
development of these children. The food and eating difficulties
may be related to the business of the parent, but this is only
speculation.

In response to questions by the housemother as to how she can
deal with present behavior, Dr. Beiser stated that housemother
can point out to Judy in her times of difficulty that she does
not seem to enjoy herself when other children do, and when she
should.

                              Mirl W. Whitaker,

D-4: LBO's Summary for Lake Bluff School—Joe

Back in the 50's Lake Bluff Orphanage sent all its residents to Lake Bluff School. It was their policy to provide the school with a summary of each child's status. This was my summary. It's interesting because it's sort of a distilled view of who I was at the time.

SUMMARY FOR LAKE BLUFF SCHOOL

Child: Joseph Thomas Blakemore

Born: July 1, 1941

Since the time of his parents first separation, five years ago, "Joey" has been living in foster homes. He has not seen his father since then. His mother has not been able to care for him because of her needing to work, but she has visited regularly each week.

Joey feels sensitive about his short height and has compensated for this by preferring the company of older boys. He wants very much to get along with the other children and has shown considerable ability to do so. He likes sports and group activities.

He is also sensitive about being one year behind in school. This resulted from his mother having him do 2nd year work over again when he had had five changes of schools during the year. His reading is poor, but his other work is average.

Grace Powers
Assistant Superintendent

JCG:vb

D-5: LBO's Summary for Lake Bluff School—Judy
This is my sister Judy's summary. As you can see, we were very different!

SUMMARY FOR LAKE BLUFF SCHOOL

Child: Judy Lynn Blakemore

Born: October 22, 1943

Since the time of her parents first separation five years ago, Judy has lived in foster homes. She has not seen her father since then. Her mother has not been able to care for her because of her needing to work, but she has visited regularly each week.

Judy tends to be poised and well mannered perhaps overly so. She is quick to express herself and may alienate other children by not being able to give ground when a difference occurs. She may prefer to play more with boys than girls and has called herself a "tomboy". She has a strong liking however, for dolls and other things of interest to girls her age.

Judy has done above average work in school and tries hard to maintain her grades.

Grace Powers

Assistant Superintendent

D-6: Letter from Caseworker re: Return of Custody to Mother

In August of 1953 my mother took the bull by the horns and decided we should be moved from LBO to my uncle's house, "without consulting" the powers that be. Is it just me, or does this letter reflect their irritation with this situation?

August 26, 1953

Mrs. Pearl A. Duncan
Probation Officer
Probation Department of Du Page County
Court House
Wheaton, Illinois

Re: Blakemore, Joseph and Judy

Dear Mrs. Duncan:

On August 17, 1953, Mrs. Ruth Blakemore asked us to return Joseph and Judy to her full custody. For the present Mrs. Blakemore is placing them with Mr. and Mrs. Kenneth Blakemore, paternal uncle and aunt. Mrs. Blakemore states that she eventually hopes to join the children in this home.

We are not acquainted with Mr. and Mrs. Kenneth Blakemore. We understand through the mother that the children are happy in their home which they share with four male cousins, ages four, six, thirteen and fifteen. Judy will share a room with the youngest boy and Joe with the three oldest.

Since Judy was making a very difficult adjustment in our institution we approve of her going into a home situation, and had in fact recommended to the mother that she cooperate with us in making a foster home placement. However, she was able to work out the above plan without our help or without consulting us.

We are therefore, recommending that the Court release us from our temporary guardianship and vacate the pay order against Mrs. Blakemore as of August 17, 1953.

Sincerely yours,

(Mrs.) Carol Hinds
Casework Supervisor

Reply Attention: Angus Sumner
CH:egd   Caseworker

257

About the Author

J.T. Blakemore lives with his wife and son in Tallahassee, Florida, where he operates a small business and continues to write. He is sixty-two years old, and Until the Cows Come Home is his first book.

Ordering Information

If you enjoyed reading this book and would like to order a copy for a friend or family member, please contact Airleaf Publishing on line at www.airleaf.com, or call them at 1-800-342-6068. We appreciate your business!